Over 50
Feeling 30!

How bioidentical hormones bring your body back

Slow and *minimize* biological aging − physically and mentally

William H. Lee, M.D.

*Lawrence
Good Friend
To your
optimal Health!
Bill*

T
TOTAL
PUBLISHING
AND MEDIA

www.TotalPublishingAndMedia.com

Book doctor: Charol Messenger, www.thewritingdoctor.biz

You are only as healthy as your most diseased part.

Dedication

This is dedicated to all those exceptional people who wish to get every drop of love, passion, happiness, and vigor out of their existence on this planet. Those of you who wish for the energy, vitality, strength, and wellness to make a difference!

Contents

The Men's Manual
Men! Recapture Your Vitality!

Conclusion

Acknowledgements

A huge thank you to my wife Sue! She is my inspiration and support. She has done so many things to help me and encourage me in completing this book (sometimes putting a burr under my saddle). She authored the inspiring opening article "One Woman's Story of *Aging Optimally!*" and has written her own books. She also has a DVD for EQ (emotional quotient) for children, which won The Parent's Choice Award and an endorsement from *Children First.* And she managed all of this while maintaining her own great health and fitness. This book would not have happened without her.

Ryan Lee did the art work. He is my son, and I am proud and happy to have his illustrations be an integral part of this book. I am grateful for his creative talent and excellent sense of humor, which lightens things up.

Thank you to Jane Anne Ferguson, who spent countless hours offering spiritual insight regarding aging and life in general. Her valuable knowledge and wisdom are included in the appendix article "A Perspective on Spiritual Aging."

Thank you to Travis Moe, in particular, who authored the appendix article "Brain Memory" regarding the important brain-mapping and cognition new medical device from WAVi. I find this groundbreaking new diagnostic tool extremely exciting. I believe it will change the way we address and understand brain health in medicine. I am so glad to introduce this new technology, and I thank Travis for his help in clearly explaining this very important new medical tool.

Lastly, a special thanks to my book doctor, Charol Messenger. She organized my extensive materials, edited with great enthusiasm, and motivated me with new ideas that have brought a greater fullness to this book for all who are seeking better health. Charol also has been a major supporter in completing this book. It would not have gotten into print without her knowledgeable assistance.

One Woman's Story of
Aging Optimally!

Really Practicing the Protocol of Age Management!

I'm Sue Lee, Dr. Lee's wife. At the time of writing this I'm sixty-one years old and I like to think I'm a good example of a healthy senior. For those who are wondering, the pictures you see here we're taken a month before I turned sixty.

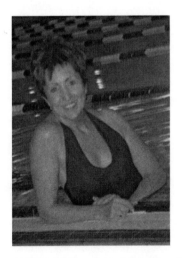

When your husband is writing a book about Age Management, people ask, "Does your wife follow this protocol? Does she do Bioidentical Hormone therapy? Does she exercise and eat a certain way?"

Bill and I thought it'd be helpful to you, the reader, to hear this from my perspective. I hope this will help you understand what it's like in the daily life of one who practices the protocol of Age Management. This comes from my heart, for I've no other way to communicate. For me, it's all about how I feel and function. I can list facts, but the bottom line for me is: Do I feel good? Am I energized? Do I feel like Me?

I'll be the first one to tell you, it isn't about a magic pill or doing short cuts. It's about living and participating in life, being aware that your health is directly correlated to how you function on a daily basis. It's easy when you're young; but somewhere along the line, lifestyle catches up and reality hits.

Is it hard to have the discipline I do? It depends upon your perspective. I think it's hard not to take care of myself, then down the line be facing a serious illness, health restrictions and operations. *That's* hard! Taking care of myself and being disciplined is worth it, for I know that what I do today will play out in my tomorrows.

So, what's it like, this Age Management thing? And what do I do to integrate wellness into my daily life?

From my perception, it is a full spirit, mind, body, and strength/energy/emotions lifestyle. I'm going to address each of these four components and give you a snapshot of what I do. If you aren't into the spirit and mind "stuff," you might skip straight to the body section, but I feel you'd be missing the most important part. It's up to you, but I hope you will stick with me and read the wholeness about wellness. After each section, I'll leave you with some questions that might help you.

My Spirit

If there is only one thing I would do, it is to take care of my spirit. For my spirit is the essence of who I am, the real *Me.*

What does this have to do with Age Management? Everything. My spirit is *who* I am housed inside my body, that people call Sue. My spirit is me having a human experience.

If my spirit is *dispirited,* it is dis-eased, out of "ease." Taking care of my spirit is the first step to my wellness.

How Do I Care for My Spirit?

What works for me may not be your choice, but might help you think about what you wish to do to be back in touch with your "spirit self" or improve upon what you are already doing.

- *First, I wake and say,* "Good Morning!" to that which is greater than I. Whatever you wish to call that (God, Universe, love, life) doesn't matter. For me, it is a connectedness I contact upon awakening. I say, "Good Morning. What might I give to the day?" For if we all give to the day, perhaps we will all get from the day.

- *I rise very early,* somewhere between 4:30 and 5:30 every day, like clockwork. I love this about myself and jokingly say that if I were a Native American, my name would be *The One Who Greets the Day.* I love waking up early and opening the day and being present with the sunlight illuminating nature and all that is around me and somehow in me.

- *I meditate* for a period of time that feels good to me. I do not turn on the television. I do not read the newspaper. I will not allow anything negative to enter my atmosphere. Is that Pollyannaish? No, I think it's smart. I then sit with a cup of coffee, as the sun rises, read a novel or self-help book, a cat upon my lap, and take time to be with Me, the person I'm going to live with my whole entire life. I am my best friend.

That's the key point here. My spirit — my Essence, ME — is the one person I will live with my whole life. For, me, that means that my essence needs to feel *good* about who she is, how she functions, what she does and what she is *feeling.*

Age Management is about that internal person feeling *great, good, alive,* and *well!* It is about honoring who I am as much as caring for the body that houses me.

I could write a whole book about just caring for our spirit. This is a chapter within this book to help you understand what I do.

Here Are Some Key Points to My Caring for My Spirit

- I try not to "sin" against my own truth. I try to communicate in thought, voice, carriage, and actions who I truly am.

- I focus on the positive as much as I can; seeing the good that is around me, and not the negative. I call myself to that task daily, over and over again.

- I smile at my own humanness and the humanness of others.

- I actually tell myself how much I like ME. I love being me and I am grateful that I get to live this life as me.

I think you're getting the point, and I won't belabor it anymore. I basically honor my spirit and feel it is significant to managing my "age." I am truly "young at heart" and I hope to maintain the wonder and awe of just being in life.

Write down:
- Where are you missing the mark? Where are you being "false" with your own truth and self?

- What concept of self do you have to let go of in order to go to the next level of self-fulfillment?

My Mind

For me, my mind is the enlivening energy that communicates with all that is around me and within me and is sometimes communicating with my brain. My mind — my viewpoint — is not my brain, but is something far greater than just that mass within my skull. My mind is an extension of my spirit and can communicate with others, with the whole of me and with all that is. My thoughts are a significant part of my mind, and that is what I'll touch on here, for it is that to which most people relate.

Thoughts.

I sit here thinking. Thoughts to me are extremely important and are the very path upon which I travel. I believe my thoughts are things and the most powerful force we humans have when used in conjunction with our feelings. Thoughts know no distance, time, or space.

I keep a positive mindset. I think positively and work at being in the "present" and "aware."

I believe that makes for healthier living, therefore a more "well" me.

I'm not dwelling on the past and not overly worrying about the future. The past has contributed powerfully to who I am, and I am forever grateful for the challenges of the past as well as the profound joys of it. I have sixty-one years of living behind me now and I find that amazing, for my mind is still focused on some of the same things that brought me joy as a child.

I believe I'm more than fairly intelligent — yet I never wanted to lose the mind of my growing-up years; the mind that focused on the sun shining upon a leaf, the scampering of a squirrel, the ripples upon the water. These things bring me joy, and joy is what I seek.

I work at being interested in the learning process, and to be interested in life and in what others are doing and are about. Yet I will not bog myself down with taking in their complaints and negativity, for I do not wish to clutter my mind with such thoughts.

If my thoughts are what create my daily life and future experience, then I wish them to be about living my best, living my fullest and living within joy.

If my thoughts are my constant companions following me daily and carrying on those constant conversations within my head, then I surely hope I can keep them companionable. Who wishes to hang out all day with a complainer? Not I. I want to be with someone fun, interested, exciting, tuned in, tapped in, and into being, into living.

So, that is where I focus and direct my thoughts.

I believe the most important conversation I ever have on any given day is the one in my own head. I love the Story People piece that says, "I once had a garden filled with ugly thoughts, but they took constant attention and one day I realized I had better things to do."[1]

When my mind is in sync with my spirit, I am more whole . . . and closer to true wellness.

Write down:

- Thoughts you wish to eliminate: _____
- *Finish this phrase:* "As of this moment, I am now working toward _____."

---

[1] www.storypeople.com/storypeople/Home.do

My Body

Ah, the body! The part most of us think about, complain about, try to tweak, manipulate. The part of us that wrinkles, gets age spots, sags, droops. Ages! Face it, gravity works — and it's doing a good job!

Where to begin when talking about the body? First, I believe we biologically have ways of functioning properly and most efficiently. So that in and of itself is important to me.

If what I put into my body affects my biology, then I'd better be aware of what I put into my mouth in order to function in a healthy way. Why? Because who I really am — the person inside, that spirit I just talked about and that mind inside me — are dependent upon my body to carry them while I live and breathe upon this Earth.

What I Eat

Whew! Under the microscope, sharing with all of you who . . . oh, my goodness . . . might judge me! I need to let go of that . . . and help you help yourself by being perfectly honest with you: I am not perfect.

People ask me, "Do you ever eat food that's bad for you?" Of course, I do. I'm human, and it's impossible to avoid some of it all the time.

I eat organic as much as I possibly can. I shop at Farmers Markets in the summer, ask if it's local, and look for organics there as well.

Breakfast

Greek yogurt, probiotics, Ezekiel 4:9 cereal, walnuts, chia seeds, fruit, one cup of coffee (my second vice, the first one is shopping); sometimes, I do teeccino coffee substitute or tea. While I eat breakfast, I read a novel or self-help book.

Lunch

Sometimes same as breakfast. Or a salad chockfull of goodies; such as greens, fruit, veggies, seeds, nuts, and one protein, with a very light dressing — very little, I like to taste the food not the dressing!

Dinner

Protein, veggie, and salad. Examples:

- Salmon, asparagus, salad
- Chicken, broccoli, salad
- Stew or soup (always homemade)

Water

Eight to ten glasses of filtered tap water a day: about three glasses in the a.m., four in the afternoon, one at night (at least two hours before bedtime).

Snacks

If I snack, it's usually a handful of nuts and/or a piece of fruit.

Alcohol

I'm not a wine drinker, never have been. If we go out, I might have one cocktail, never two.

Desserts

If we go out and we both feel like having dessert, we share one.

Yes, sometimes I love a burger, with bacon, cheese, mushrooms, and fries. Not often, but enough to know I'm human. And it tastes good! Like an ice-cream cone on a hot summer day brings back wonderful childhood memories.

Supplements I Take After Breakfast

- Antioxidant (Nutrilite brand)

- Two concentrated fruits and vegetables (Nutrilite brand)

- Multi-vitamin (Nutrilite's Double X) — 3 tablets: one minerals, one vitamins, one phytonutrients; the latter are minute nutrients that plants develop to protect themselves from disease, draught, insects, poisons. I figure that if they're good for the plants and we eat those plants, they're good for us. Which is exactly what has been discovered!

- 4 vitamin C, 250 mg each — I choose these over a single 1,000 mg, because I know and trust the brand Nutrilite and that's the size it comes in.

- 2 vitamin B complex (Nutrilite brand)

- 7 capsules omega 3 (total of 4,000 mg EPA and 1,400 mg DHA)

- 1 lutein (Nutrilite brand) — Supports healthy eyes. Contains a unique blend of bilberry, marigold, black currant, spinach, and vitamin.

- 1 CoQ10, 30 mg (Nutrilite brand) — Makes energy for our heart cells to do their work. As we age, our enzyme levels drop.

- 1 potassium, 99 mg — Works in conjunction with magnesium to lower blood pressure.

- 1 magnesium, 150 mg — For blood pressure and sleep. The most used mineral in the body.

- 1 vitamin K, 100 mcg — Drives calcium to the bone.

- 1 curcumin, 750 mg — Many known benefits, including: inhibition and prevention of some cancers, cardiovascular support, antioxidant, and anti-inflammatory.

- 1 rhodiola, 200 mg — Owes its healing powers to being an adaptogen, meaning it helps the body adapt to and resist stressful conditions, such as depression, sleep deprivation, toxins.

- 1 NAC, 600 mg — This is the stable form of the amino acid cysteine. It is a powerhouse of a supplement with potent antioxidant activity. In addition to combating exercise-induced damage to muscle tissue, it helps to detoxify the liver, build connective tissue, fight viral infections, and combat the effects of age. NAC turns into glutathione, which is the "master antioxidant"; and it helps to metabolize estrogen. And these are only the highlights!

- 3 lecithin — This fatlike substance, called a phospholipid, is needed by every cell in the body and is a key building block of cell membranes. It aids in clarifying the brain and memory.

- ½ clondine — This is a pharmaceutical product for blood pressure.

- 1 spironolactone — This is a pharmaceutical product for blood pressure and mild diuretic.

Bedtime Supplements
- 3 vitamin C, 250 mg

- 1 potassium, 99 mg

- 1 magnesium, 150 mg

- 1 combination calcium-magnesium, 250 calcium/100 magnesium — Adds bone support.

- ½ clondine — For blood pressure.

- 1 spironolactone — For blood pressure.

- 1 sublingual vitamin D (3000 IU) — Under my tongue until it absorbs.

- 1 melatonin pill, 1 mg — For sleep. Melatonin is secreted into the blood by the *pineal gland* in the brain and decreases as we age. It's a major brain antioxidant.

WEIGHT – The Dreaded "W" Word!

Winter of eighth grade, I weighed 179 pounds and I'm small-boned, really. To figure this, you go by your wrist measurement. I'm 5'7" and my wrist is 5.5". Here's the chart:

Female Wrist Measurements

Height less than 5' 2" (Less than 155cms)	Height 5' 2" - 5' 5" (155cms - 163cms)	Height more than 5' 5" (More than 163cms)
Less than 5.5" (140mm)	Less than 6.0" (152mm)	Less than 6.25" (159mm)
5.5" - 5.75" (140 - 146mm)	6" - 6.25" (152 - 159mms)	6.25" - 6.5" (159 - 165mm)
More than 5.75" (146mm)	More than 6.25" (159mm)	More than 6.5" (165mm)

I didn't like what I weighed. With the love and support of my mother, I lost fifty pounds. She said I had to do it in a healthy way —

by eating a balanced diet and exercising. It took me three weeks initially to lose two pounds. Then I lost two pounds every week!

I loved how I felt and looked after that — so I kept at it. I was very disciplined, and I began teaching aerobics to a handful of friends. Then I taught aerobics in an organized fashion for thirty-six years.

I am not naturally thin. I've worked at it. I believe we are creatures of movement and that we should *move.*

At the age of fifty-six, I quit teaching aerobics, yet I maintained the same workout schedule. However, two years later, I had gained twenty pounds! I was shocked! The "fat" around the middle, which creeps in with women during menopause, had found me! I was shocked! I had worked so hard!

Faced with a cortisol-expanded trunk, waist and thighs, I said to my husband, Dr. Lee, "When you can figure out how to help women lose this fat, you will be every woman's best friend!" Fat was *not* going to be my story!

I am now sixty-one — and I have lost sixteen of those pounds that crept in. I feel good, look great, and I function with energy and vitality. I now weigh 135 on a regular basis.

How Did I Do It?

- Dr. Lee did adjust my *thyroid,* which was low.

- *Hormones* have to be balanced in order to lose weight. I believe that taking Estrogen Balance helped to detoxify my estrogen hormonal system. (I use Vital Nutrients' Estrogen Balance.)

- I followed the *Glycemic Index* (see appendix, as well as "Sugar Overload" in chapter two: *To Reduce Your Glycation*).

- *I exercised!* Movement, weights, stretching, core balance and stabilization, as described next.

- Recently I detoxed, using Metagenics' Ultra Clear for shakes and their Advaclear capsule, and I lost an additional five pounds!

Exercise!

It's not about over-exercising, which actually can age you. Here's what worked for me: Doing something physical every day.

I keep the same routine I always have: not overly aerobic, but *consistent.*

Movement / Aerobic

- *In good weather, I walk daily* — three to seven miles, which takes me about two hours for six miles, for it's very hilly where we live. I walk with walking poles (Nordic All4Walk, www.all4walk.com), which help with posture; utilizing upper body and burning calories (burns about 20% more calories).

- *Monday, Wednesday, Friday* — If not walking, I ride my indoor stationary bike forty to sixty minutes.

- I also run in water on a regular basis in my local gymnasium pool. The depth is three-and-a-half feet the entire length of the pool, which works well for running. Water is twelve times the resistance of air, and it's a phenomenal workout! I've been running in water for over twenty years, and I often will be in the pool rather than doing the bike or walking.

Weight Lifting

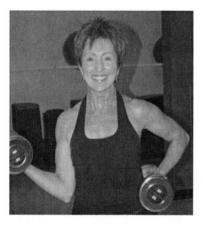

Tuesday, Thursday, Saturday — I lift weights. Why? Muscle burns fat.

We lose muscle rapidly as we age — if we aren't rebuilding it. We have to develop muscle . . . and maintain it.

I do two sets of twelve for each of these below (which is not overdoing it).

- *Leg press.* I warm-up with two 45-pound weights. Then I add two more 45-pound weights and do another set of twelve. I sometimes do very, very slow repetitions — two inch drop with the bar, and hold for a count of thirty; two more inches, hold etc.; returning up the same way.

- *Leg extension quads* (50 pounds, two sets of twelve). Again, I sometimes do two-inch increments, holding each time to a count of thirty or so, then up another two inches, etc.

- *Leg curls hamstrings.* I use a machine that has separate leg capability, and I do fifteen pounds with each leg.

- *Lateral pull downs* (60 pounds)

- *Pectoral machine* (chest muscles) (50 pounds)

- *Deltoids* (15 pounds)

- *Biceps* (15 pounds)

- *Triceps* (25 pounds)

At times, I incorporate other weight activities. Following are the basics I always do:

Stretching

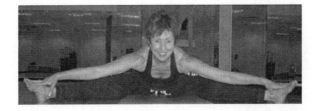

Tuesday, Thursday, Saturday — after the weights: I s-t-r-e-t-c-h. I cannot emphasize this enough!

If you haven't noticed it, your muscles have probably gotten very tight. Tight muscles are a major contributor to an unbalanced core, accidental falls, and not being able to prevent or regain balance once a fall begins.

Flexibility helps with overall range of motion around joints and the muscles, so they work together to accomplish the tasks they're called upon to do. As we age, our movements become restricted, which totally affects our whole quality of life.

Stretching should be done regularly — and with patience.

Ease into it. Do not bounce. Do not go to the point where a muscle quivers; quivering muscles on a stretch is not good. Do not go to the point of pain.

But do s-t-r-e-t-c-h. You're worth it, and the functionality of your daily life is worth it!

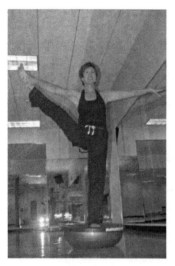

Fluidity of movement disguises aging as well as anything else! I don't move like an old lady.

Core Balance and Stabilization

Yes, this is me on a half ball, showing off. Why? Because it makes me feel good. It feels good that I'm still flexible enough to stretch my leg out and strong enough that I can balance on one foot — while doing so on a half ball.

I work at balance. Balance is directly related to our core strength and must be developed and maintained. As we age, balance goes quickly — and you find yourself feeling old without it.

Our core is commonly known as our center of gravity. This is basically the area around the trunk and pelvis. A strong core assists in the balance of our body, overall stabilization, and support to the back. I actually practice balancing, with standing on one foot doing various movements.

To do balance work, we utilize our core and strengthen it. It's important to notice such things as the articulation of your feet and being tuned into the work your feet are doing.

Try standing on one foot, with the other foot bent 90 degrees and elevated waist high (if you can get it there).

Then pay attention to what your supportive leg's foot and ankle are doing. They are probably moving quite a bit . . . and it's important that they can and do. Our feet do a tremendous job in supporting our body. Try this:

- Stand on one foot. Hold. Switch legs.

- Stand up on your toes. Drop down.

  - Put one leg out behind you.

  - Drop down on the supporting leg.

  - Feel that trembling in your thigh.

- Feel your foot working to keep you in place, the articulation of your ankle.

- Use those crazy-looking balance disc pillows (soft flexible round, folks use them in gyms). They work!

Write down:

- For my body I now will _____.
- The three new steps I'm taking for my body, because I'm worth it: _____

- _____.

Posture

Okay, I'm finally going to have my say about posture, something I've always wanted to say.

People, stand up! Too many of you are walking around with your shoulders slumped, tummies sticking out, lower backs curved, heads jutted out and down.

We are not meant to stand like that! We are meant to *stand up,* to look around and be aware of our environment.

Yet I see so many people walking around like the weight of the world is literally on their shoulders.

If you have to fool yourself into feeling good, then do so. *Stand tall.* Walk like you're important and that you have some place to be going.

Am I sometimes tired? You bet — but when I'm walking, I stand up, abs tight and shoulders back — and I *stride*.

If you walk like life is weighing you down, believe me it will and, someday, it will take you down.

I hope, to the day I die, that I walk with purpose and interest in what is around me.

Strength > Energy > Emotions

Putting it all together — spirit, mind, body — gives me my *functional strength*.

My energy level results from my emotions. When I care for myself — paying attention to my spirit, my mind, and my body, having these three in sync and working together — I have an *energy* that feels so right, so ME! My emotional barometer then is so "on," so in the groove and so how I wish to feel and be!

Strength > Energy > Emotions get us through the day. Be focused *on* the day. Be *within* the day.

Too many people at day's end think, "Thank God I got through it again." Shame on us. What have we done to ourselves? It isn't about surviving the day. It's about *thriving* within the day. You don't have to be a dynamo, but wouldn't it be wonderful if you felt like *living* the day — really *present* with it?

Write down:

My strength > energy > emotions check-up:

- Where am I with my Spiritual strength/energy/emotions? _____

- Where am I with my Mind strength/energy/emotions? _____

- Where am I with my Body strength/energy/emotions? _____

- Where am I with my strength/energy/emotions? _____

- Where do I wish to be? _____

Bioidentical Hormone Therapy

This is the fine-tuning of taking care of my body in a comprehensive wellness program. I feed and efficiently "nutritionalize" my body so the hormones can work properly. The hormones have to be the proper ones for my body, the ones identical to the biological structure of my body. To honor who I am — my spirit, my mind, my body, my strength/energy/emotions — I take care of the hormonal component of aging . . . to live well!

Dr. Lee looks at my blood levels, and we work on what works for *my* body. I've been on hormone supplementation since I was thirty-eight and bioidentical hormones since age fifty-one.

What are the benefits? For me, they are many:

- I'm not as fatigued as my friends.
- I have physical endurance.
- I'm more toned.
- My brain is clear, and my memory is working.
- My skin is not as wrinkled.
- My stomach is flatter.
- I'm mentally sharp and alert.
- Foggy brain is a thing of the past.
- I don't have night sweats.
- I don't have hot flashes.
- Sex is still a loving activity.
- Life feels worth living.
- I face the day with excitement and enthusiasm!

Hormonally I use:

- Estrogen patch. I've been on hormone therapy since age thirty-eight and bioidentical since 1999. I trust my diet and other aspects of what I do for my body. I know that I probably would be in worse health if I did not take estrogen.
- Progesterone in a capsule
- Testosterone in a cream
- DHEA in a tablet

- Thyroid tablet.

Age Management, for me, is not just having a good-looking body but a *functioning* one. It is about having my spirit, mind, and body working together to provide me with the strength, energy, and emotional harmony to be a participant in life.

I believe that life is what we participate in, not what happens to us. To participate in my own health of spirit, mind, body, strength, energy, and emotions allows me to be the heroine in my own life story. At day's end, I am aware that I *thrived* instead of merely survived — which is knowing I lived my life as if it matters, for it does!

I hope what I have shared with you will help you help yourself to be more disciplined — not because you have to be, but because you wish it for yourself.

This is your life. It's not too late to begin living well.

Everything I do for myself results in the combined components of who I am. They are not separate. Someday, my body will separate from who I am. I will leave it, and I will thank it for carrying me so well for so many years.

– Sue Lee (2010)

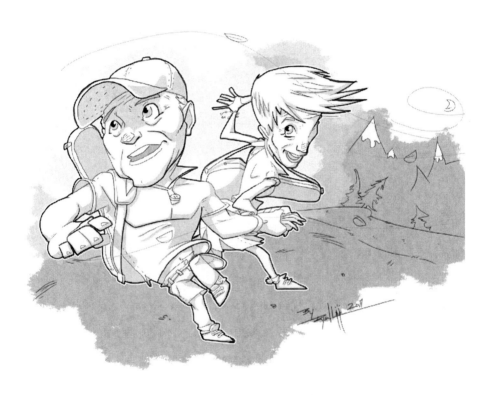

Illustration by Ryan Lee

How to Get

Your Body Back!

Introduction

Remember the energy of your youth? You could run and play all day and never get tired? Remember how you never seemed to gain weight, no matter how many malts, fries, or cheese burgers you ate? Remember how you were able to stay up late at parties and it didn't affect how you felt the next day? Remember how smooth and firm your skin used to be?

The body ages by becoming diseased. In this book, I tell you how to get your body back, how to look and feel decades younger.

Your *chronological* age is how many years you have lived. Your *biological* age is certain parts of the body wearing out faster than others; due to viruses, bacteria, toxins, poor nutrition, lack of exercise, trauma (physical or emotional), etc. For example, someone who develops heart disease or plaque in the blood vessels "ages" the heart. A fifty-five year old *chronologically* could have a heart that is seventy-five years old *biologically*. Is that you?

The good news is we all can do many things to improve our *biological* age. My mother had it right all along. "Eat right, get plenty of sleep, and avoid things that hurt you" (like smoking, drinking alcohol, eating too much sugar). To detour away from disease toward good health, we need to exercise and manage our stress, make healthy food choices, and take supplements and hormones. Some people work with a life coach to help them with this commitment, through accountability.

Exercise is key to optimal health and needs to be consistent; working with a trainer can help you get started right. Proper *nutrition* is paramount, and working with a nutritionist is helpful in the beginning. Getting enough *sleep* is priceless for reducing stress. *Total hormonal balance* is critical for long-term and overall health; for this, you *do* need a physician who is knowledgeable.[2]

Hormones are essential to the body. They are needed for health, energy, well-being, and running the body's normal processes. Hormone replenishment is *very* necessary. There have been a lot of studies, both pro and con, about hormone replacement therapy. I recommend *bioidentical* hormones, because they are biologically, atom to atom, the same as what the human body produces. They are safe, effective and, in fact, needed.

The human body is a miraculous machine. It repairs itself. For many years, it puts up with insults like tobacco and alcohol, over-exercise, and lack of sleep. However, like water wearing away rock to

---

[2]   Check out the American Association of Anti-Aging Medicine website, www.worldhealth.net. You can find an Age Management doctor or practitioner in your area at their directory. Most listed are doing cosmetic procedures like lasers, acid peals, and dermabrasion; however, some M.D.s listed are knowledgeable about nutrition, exercise, and bioidentical hormone replacement. Other websites include www.SuzanneSomers.com, www.LifeExtension.com, and www.FunctionalMedicine.org.

form a canyon in a mountain, these forces eventually take their toll on the body and wear it down. Any machine, even well-maintained, eventually wears out.

Twelve major forces affect our health, memory, mood, and sanity: inflammation, sugar overload, free radicals, impaired natural detoxification, blood clots, stress, insufficient nutrition, insufficient exercise, shortening of our DNA telomeres, insufficient hormones (both men and women), deficiency in our human growth hormone, and deficiency in our brain neurotransmitters.

We all age, but at different rates. In the following pages, I define how each of these twelve physical conditions causes aging — *and* how to *slow* and *minimize* unhealthy life patterns. You want to keep everything working: eyes, ears, brain, heart, joints, immune system, and sexual function. That is how to remain vital and without the chronic degenerative diseases typically associated with aging.

I wholeheartedly welcome you into these pages of self-discovery — to help you get your body back! To take charge of your wellness — because I know it can be done.

The 12 Causes of Aging

and

How to *Minimize* Them!

1

Inflammation

Inflammation is actually part of the body's defense system. The immune system utilizes inflammation to protect us from bacteria, viruses, toxins, and other infections, even splinters; and seeks to rid us of abnormal cell growth, called cancer. Another part of the inflammatory response is to clean up debris from the battle waged by the immune system to promote healing.

So, inflammation can be a very good thing. However, in today's society with our rush – rush lifestyle, most of us have turned on this system to the extreme and we have way too much inflammation. A common way it shows up is in joint aches and pains and a general overall feeling of malady, whose origin is difficult to identify. Most often, the damage is going on undetected, without any symptoms until it is too late. This excessive inflammation is the number one problem facing overweight, sedentary Americans.

Excessive inflammation over decades can result in many adverse symptoms and illnesses, none of which we would choose. Inflammation is associated with diabetes, cancer, joint disease, and bone loss (deterioration). It can lead to America's number one killer, heart disease. It can cause the most feared disease, dementia. Which of these would you like to have?

Inflammation can age us prematurely. It is a core issue with numerous chronic degenerative diseases; such as, heart disease, cancer, high blood pressure, stroke, diabetes, joint disease, dementia, and anything ending in "itis," like colitis, sinusitis, arthritis.

When in excess, our inflammatory "soldiers" (cytokines, interleukins, leukotrienes, NFkbeta, tumor necrosis factor) don't have enough "bad guys" to destroy and they begin destroying the body, instead; such as, the protective membranes in our joints, our brain cells involved with memory, and the vascular linings that initiate plaque formation (atherosclerotic plaque or hardening of the arteries); plaque forms with elevated cholesterol or sugar or triglycerides.

Also, the more inflammation we have, the more cortisol is called upon to "put out the fire." Cortisol is a hormone the body releases in response to inflammation. It stops the major destructive part of inflammation and initiates a healing process. This is essential day in and day out. However, because of all the tremendous stress we experience daily in the modern world, we tend to have too much cortisol. In excess, cortisol can be very destructive. It tears down muscles, ligaments, and bones — *and* puts on fat.

Causes of Inflammation

1. *Sugar*

The number one cause of excessive inflammation today is excessive sugar intake. In 1800, the average American consumed only 2 to 4 pounds in one year. In the standard modern American diet, the average person consumes 167 pounds of sugar in one year — or a half pound *every* day!

We still have basically the same body, the same metabolism, and the same amount of insulin as the human body always did. The body simply cannot keep up with ingesting this much sugar. It spikes the insulin level, resulting in all the symptoms and effects of inflammation. After a few years, diabetes follows.

Sadly, many youths consume 50 to 60 percent of their calories as refined sugar and high fructose corn syrup. Even more worrisome than the calories consumed is that the enormous quantities of sugar turn on the unhealthy parts of our genes, injuring the body's cells and organs. When we consume sugar, insulin is released to deal with it. Elevated insulin increases inflammation, and the body's normal response to inflammation is to elevate cortisol . . . which makes us fat.

Insulin and Insulin Resistance

What is insulin? It's simply a hormone, made in the pancreas. Its function is to transport glucose (sugar) from the blood stream into the cells. The sugar, or fat, then goes to the mitochondria, where it is transformed into energy via a series of complex chemical reactions called the Krebs Cycle, where ATP is made.

ATP is what our body uses for energy. It's the "fuel" to our body like gasoline is to a car. Our "fuel" can be made from glucose or fat, sometimes, as a last resort, even protein. Our body is intended to be a fat burner, primarily; glucose is reserved for emergency boosts. However, in our current civilization, we have become glucose burners, instead; which is causing numerous health problems. The high levels of glucose make us fat, promote atherosclerosis and heart disease, and increase inflammation; thereby, triggering the chronic degenerative diseases of "aging."

Insulin also helps to transport amino acids (constituents of protein) into cells. This allows our body's cells to promote healing; which occurs after exercise, for example. When we eat a constant diet of too many carbohydrates (which become glucose), we are forcing our pancreas to pour out more and more insulin to normalize the level of glucose in the blood stream. Frequently, we are not getting enough protein. (As a gross generalization, women eat too many carbs and not enough protein.)

When this sugar load goes on and on, day after day, year after year, eventually the interaction between the insulin and the insulin receptor on the cell membrane becomes sluggish and doesn't work well. We come to a point where, although we have enough insulin, the response is slowed and the sugar level in the blood stream remains too high. This is "insulin resistance," or Type 2 Diabetes. In other words, we have too high a level of glucose, too high a level of insulin, and our cells are "starved" for glucose to make more energy. The entire system becomes dysfunctional.

Because we have too high a level of glucose, the pancreas must make even more insulin, which leads to the inflammation and chronic diseases of aging (heart disease, cancer, diabetes, dementia, joint disease). If this continues for a long time, the pancreas becomes exhausted and cannot keep up, meaning there is too little insulin for normalizing the blood sugar. This is full-blown Type 1 diabetes.

2. *Food Allergies*

The second leading cause of inflammation is hidden food allergies; especially dairy, soy, egg, and wheat gluten.

Gluten is part of all grains (e.g., wheat, rye, barley, oats). It is a molecule to which some people are allergic. Allergy symptoms may include: stomach cramps, gas, bloating, indigestion, headaches, feeling poorly, depression, weight gain.

Gluten is in many, many foods that Americans commonly eat. There are many books and cookbooks about how to eat gluten-free; gluten-free foods also may be found at health-food stores. Multiple articles on gluten and gluten allergy are available online.

The best way to figure out if you are gluten sensitive is to go without it for six weeks and see how you feel. This is not an easy task, but it may pay you big dividends.

Many people are unaware of their food allergies and sensitivities, and unaware of the dire consequences in health maladies. Part of this is because sometimes there is a delayed reaction of one or two days after eating the offending food, which makes it difficult to identify the allergy source.

When we start reacting to one or two foods, our immune system becomes hyped up. Then we may start reacting to many foods; however, these are secondary reactions and may be sensitivities rather than true allergies. The difference is sensitivities can revert to normal once the immune system gets a chance to rest and calm down, which may take three to six months.

Left unchecked, true allergies invoke an inflammatory reaction continually. After a decade or two, this can lead to the consequences of inflammation: heart disease, diabetes, hypertension, cancer, dementia, joint disease.

3. *Fat*

The third greatest cause of inflammation is fat accumulation. Fat puts out hormones and cytokins, which are injurious to the body.

Two-thirds of the U.S. population are overweight (generally 20 pounds above the current recommended weight for the height; usually measured by the body mass index, or BMI). One-third are obese (generally 30 pounds over the ideal weight for the height; many draw the line at a BMI of 30). For the first time ever, adult life expectancy has dropped instead of going up gradually year after year.

Our children are more obese than ever recorded, increasingly more so year by year. Because of the childhood obesity epidemic, for the first time in American history our children will not live as many years as their parents will live. Children also are getting diseases that previously were seen only in adults: hypertension, diabetes, joint disease, even heart disease. These are all inflammation and fat-related.

Your waist-to-hip ratio is a good personal guide. According to the national guidelines, a woman's waist should be less than 35 inches (optimal is less than 30 inches). A man's waist should be less than 40 inches (optimal is less than 35 inches).

In my opinion, we *all* need to get away from the TV and computer and play hard *physically.* We need to eat whole foods and avoid highly refined and prepared foods, which are digested as sugar. This step alone can reduce the life-long cost of medical care dramatically and create a healthier life.

To give Americans a strong incentive, I support new thinking in which people's insurance premiums would reflect their health; perhaps something like premiums going up 1 percent per pound overweight. This is fair, because the people with excess weight consume many more healthcare services: heart stents, by-pass surgeries, cancer surgery and treatments, joint replacements, and care for the demented. These are all very expensive — and are mostly avoidable. This idea has some rough edges and needs refinement, but I think it is worth evaluation.

4. *Stress*

Another common cause of inflammation is stress; whether it is emotional, overwork, physical (over-exercise), gut issues, food allergies, intestinal or parasitic infection, toxins, or lack of sleep, etc.

For more on how stress ages you, and how better to manage it, see "Cause of Aging 6, Stress."

To Reduce Inflammation

1. *Reduce Sugar*

Reducing high-glycemic sweeteners and foods is extremely important. One low-glycemic *natural* sweetener is agave nectar, found in local health-food stores near the honeys. One patient's blood sugar had risen by ten points in one year, from 99 to 109, higher than it had ever registered. At her next annual blood test, her blood sugar had dropped to 89, *below* the previous level; she only had replaced her coffee sweetener (honey) with the mild-tasting, low-glycemic agave nectar.

A good *artificial* sweetener is stevia, derived from a plant. However, most artificial sweeteners are not healthy, and it's best to avoid them. *Equal* and others still create a rise in insulin and may have adverse effects on the brain in some sensitive individuals. Another artificial sweetener is the sugar alcohol, Xylitol.

2. *Remove Foods to Which You Are Allergic*

First, determine what food allergies you have. This may require allergy testing with a knowledgeable doctor. There are various ways to do this testing and various measurements that can be taken: IgA, IgE, IgG, IgM.

Once the allergies are identified (for example, that you are allergic to milk), all you have to do is completely remove all milk products from your diet. This may be easier said than done, but it is exceedingly important to your current and long-term health. You will be rewarded in how much better you feel!

3. *Lose Weight*

Losing weight helps *every* health marker in the body. It's critical to your overall health.

The primary steps to weight loss are:

- Increase activity.

- Decrease sugar.

- Work with the Glycemic Index (see appendix). It charts the glycemic level of many foods, and identifies how rapidly the various carbohydrates turn into sugar in the body.

- Detoxify your body (see chapter four "Impaired Natural Detoxification").

For reaching your optimal weight, in the chapter "Cause of Aging 8" see the section "Your Optimal Body Weight."

4. *Exercise Daily*

Some form of regular, moderate exercise can reduce inflammation by reducing stress and burning off extra sugar, cholesterol, and fat. You should exercise daily, getting your heart rate elevated for twenty to thirty minutes.

(*Note:* Over-exercise actually can increase inflammation.)

For how insufficient exercise causes aging and how much exercise you really need, see "Cause of Aging 8: Insufficient Exercise."

5. Take Omega 3 Fish Oil Supplement

Omega 3 is an anti-inflammatory. Dr. Barry Sears, author of the *Anti-Inflammation Zone Diet* and the *Zone Diet*, recommends that the average American take 3,000 mg daily of a combination of DHA and EPA omega 3. When there are concerns of inflammation in the body, the dose may be increased safely up to 10,000 mg daily.

For more on the benefits of omega 3s, see "Good Fat" in the section "Optimal Nutrition—To Fuel the Body" in the chapter "Cause of Aging 7: Insufficient Nutrition."

6. Take Vitamin D₃ Supplement

Vitamin D actually functions like a hormone, and it is anti-inflammatory. You can have your current level of vitamin D in your blood stream measured with a simple blood test. I have found that 98 percent of my patients are deficient and need the supplement. The amount varies from person to person, but most people need 2,000 to 10,000 units daily. Because vitamin D is fat soluble, you need to have your levels in the blood stream measured and followed by your physician, so that you do not become toxic.

7. *Take Curcumin Supplement*

Part of the spice turmeric, curcumin is now recognized as a major anti-inflammatory, as well as antioxidant and anticancer fighter. It's difficult to get enough from eating curry. It's easy to take one capsule a day.

Curcumin also aids in wound healing. It's miraculous!

The spices rosemary and ginger also reduce inflammation.

8. *Take One Low-Dose Aspirin Daily*

Often called "baby" aspirin, the dose of 81 mg once a day is recommended by many medical doctors. I have found that 200 mg daily of Advil is also very effective.

Simple Lab Tests

The following six simple, common lab tests can identify whether your poor health symptoms are due to high inflammation, so you may more immediately and effectively treat the ailment.

- *Fasting Insulin*

  High insulin is a serious problem in the United States. At least one-third of Americans have diabetes, a disease in which the person typically has very high insulin levels (until the pancreas "burns out" and the diabetic has to take insulin because the body no longer can produce enough on its own).

  Elevated insulin is inflammatory. This inflammation may increase heart disease, dementia, and vascular disease; knock out the kidneys, cause blindness. Some physicians are starting to call dementia "Type 3 Diabetes."

  So it is critical to have your fasting insulin level tested in a lab. A simple blood test will determine whether you are at risk for diabetes.

  HgbA1c is another good way to see what your average blood sugar has been over the past two to three months. An elevated result may indicate diabetes which, as explained above, is an inflammatory condition.

- *Allergy Tests*

  Hidden food allergies are the second most common cause of inflammation. When people have an allergic reaction of any kind, it sets off an inflammatory response. Testing the immune globulins (Ig) helps to check an immune system already in high gear. Common allergy tests are the IgA, IgG, or IgE. These are usually blood tests; although some doctors still do the old skin tests.

There is a newer test (LEAP) that measures your own blood cells against different potential allergens, which allows the doctors to see the direct response to individual foods. The LEAP test can check ninety-two different foods and spices.

There is also the similar ALCAT testing. They can test for 100s of foods, spices, colors, and additives.

The simplest treatment is to eliminate the offending food(s) from your diet.

- *C Reactive Protein* (CRP)

    Age Management doctors and progressive cardiologists frequently use the "hsCRP" (highly sensitive C Reactive Protein) test to measure inflammation. We also look for the cause of the inflammation. If the C Reactive Protein is elevated, you may need anti-inflammatories; such as fish oil, vitamin D, and/or curcumin. For predicting heart disease, this is as important as measuring LDL cholesterol, or measuring homocysteine.

- *Il-6 (interleukin 6)*

    This compound released during an inflammatory reaction is measureable. Elevation signifies that a lot of inflammation is actively occurring in the body. As this is not typically tested, except by Age Management doctors, you need to request it.

- *Anti-nuclear Antibody*

    Antibodies are useful against viruses and bacteria. However, in excess, patients may develop an auto-immune disease, such as Lupus or Scleroderma, in which the immune system has turned against itself. Testing your immune system can determine whether you have elevated antibodies that are working against your body's healthy cells. This is an antibody that is attacking the nucleus of your own cells!

- *Omega 3 & 6 Fatty Acids*

    This great test is just now becoming more mainstream. Since Omega 3s are generally anti-inflammatory, and Omega 6s are generally inflammatory, some cutting-edge doctors are now measuring the levels in blood of these fatty acids to help determine one's state of inflammation or need for more Omega 3. Most of us are deficient in Omega 3s, and have an over-abundance of Omega 6s.

To Reduce the Risk of Cancer

"You have cancer." These are some of the most frightening words anyone can hear. Cancer is growing in the U.S. and throughout the world. It is on the verge of being the leading cause of death in the United States, overtaking heart disease.

We live in a very toxic world. We are exposed to radiation and thousands of chemicals, pesticides, herbicides, petrochemicals, and heavy metals. Our diets are woefully inadequate and our nutrition is poor. Even though we have plentiful food sources in the United States, many foods are nutrient-deprived . . . and are literally "starving" our bodies. It is paradoxical that some people may be obese yet be starving at the same time.

A starving, nutrient-deprived body has a toxic overload and is dealing with too much inflammation; mainly from too much sugar and insufficient restorative exercise and hormones. This is a body with a compromised immune system, shutting down. It's like storming the beach at Normandy without a gun or body armor, wearing bright red and yelling, "You can't hit me." Your body gets the brunt of the attack. You feel it in poor health.

Reverse Your Inflammation

We are easy targets for cancer. To reduce the risk of cancer, reverse your inflammation. Here is what you need:

- *Optimal Nutrition* — Fuel to fight back

- *Decreased refined sugar* — To fight inflammation and reduce weight

- *Vegetables and fruits* (10 servings daily, fist sized) — To strengthen your immune system soldiers and increase the protective phytonutrients.

- *Supplements for your body's natural detoxification process* — High dose B vitamins and folic acid, trimethyl glycine, MSM, SAMe, NAC, glutamine, curcumin, alpha lipoic acid, grape seed extract, green tea, Schizandra berry, glutathione. Many of these can be found in various products called something like "Detox Formula."

- *Supplements to fight inflammation* — Omega 3s, increased vitamin D, curcumin, ASA (acetylsalicylic acid; i e., aspirin)

- *Supplements to boost your immune system* — DHEA, vitamin D, curcumin, green tea, probiotics (good bacteria for intestines)

- *Lowered cortisol* — By decreasing insulin, eliminating foods to which you are allergic, decreasing fat, decreasing stress

- *Antioxidants* — Vitamins C and E and multi-carotenes (part of vitamin A) (there are many, many others)

- *Weight loss* — Mainly by reducing sugar via the Glycemic Index (see appendix)

- *Consistent exercise*

- *Total hormonal balance* — With bioidentical hormones

- *No smoking*

- *No alcohol*

- *Lower-fat diet* (low trans fats, low saturated fats)

Unlike popular fad diets, some fat is actually good for us. Fat makes us feel satiated and slows digestion (slows glucose absorption). In terms of energy, there is about three times more energy in fat compared to sugar or protein.

We do need to avoid trans fats and saturated fats — but polyunsaturated fatty acids (PUFAs) are needed for the brain and to insulate our nerves; as well as for cell membranes, where hormone receptors reside and molecules need to flow easily into and out of the cells.

PUFAs are the omega 3, 6, and 9 fats. Omega 6s (abundant in vegetable oils and animal fats) are mostly inflammatory and do need to be avoided. However, omega 3s are anti-inflammatory; Omega 3s come mainly from fish, some from flax seed. Fish oils (omega 3) are twenty times better for the human body compared to flax seed oil, because fish oil is closer to what the body needs; flax seeds are, however, a good protein and a good fiber. Omega 9s are also healthy; they come from nuts, seeds, and avocadoes. So, we need not be afraid of all fats: Omega 3s and 9s are good for us!

- *Alkaline diet.*

    Generally speaking, vegetables and fruits are more alkaline; protein is more acidic. There is some evidence that cancer thrives better in an acidic environment and is inhibited in an alkaline environment.

    However, I have a problem with accepting the theory that an alkaline diet will inhibit cancer. The human body has intricate and abundant mechanisms for maintaining a very narrow range of pH (acid/alkaline balance). So, it is difficult for me to believe that eating specific foods will affect the pH balance in our body, either positively or negatively.

    Some people are *selling* alkaline water. Water is H_2O. OH is alkaline. H by itself and not balanced is acidic. Neither OH nor H exists in any quantity, or for any length of time, in water. H_2O *cannot* be alkaline without adding some kind of salt or mineral. If it were either acidic or alkaline, the body's pH balance mechanism quickly would reverse it to a normal human pH of 7.4.

    Get your alkaline pH in the foods you eat. Water is free.

Inflammation underlies the daily lives of most Americans. If inflammation has influenced our health and genes for two or three

29

decades, one or more of the chronic degenerative diseases of "aging" then will be diagnosed; and we'll have to battle *that* disease with all sorts of unwanted medications, tests, and therapies, which are expensive. Avoidance of these diseases is relatively inexpensive.

One of the greatest reasons for the high cost of health care is that few people are taking care of themselves. One of the greatest ways to secure a healthy retirement is to stay healthy, so you avoid a diagnosis you do not want!

2

Sugar Overload

(Glycation)

*B**eing overweight is diabetes waiting to happen!*
Sugar overload is one of the most severe health problems in America, and it is becoming a worldwide problem.

Too much sugar in the blood is associated with diabetes. Sugar overload is associated with "glycation." Even before diabetes is recognized, *glycation* is going on. Prior to that insulin levels are too high. This means that sugar is *abnormally* attaching to proteins, which creates "cross bridging" and AGEs (Advanced Glycolated End products) that gum up the works, keeping the body from performing optimally. This is a huge problem in the U.S., where two-thirds of the people are overweight and one-third are obese and diabetic (and half of those don't know it).

Sugar Overload Is Glycation

Glycation is the pathological process of a sugar molecule attaching to a protein. Hemoglobin is a protein. When sugar attaches to hemoglobin, it results in glycolated hemoglobin — which accelerates aging and can be a very serious health problem. Excessive glycation leads to plaque, fat, and the maladies of diabetes; including blindness, peripheral neuropathy, kidney disease and failure, heart disease, and dementia.

You can measure your glycation level with the simple blood test, Hemoglobin A1c (HgbA1c). An elevated HgbA1c indicates that one has had high glucose levels for at least two months. This also correlates to elevated insulin levels over a long period. An optimal HgbA1c level is 5.3. Many people have higher levels. A level greater than 6.0 is considered Type 2 Diabetes; which usually can be reversed with a big reduction in sugar and carbohydrate intake, by following the Glycemic Index in food choices (see appendix). Exercise is one of the best ways to lower blood sugar and long-term to reduce the HgbA1c.

Remember, insulin is inflammatory and leads to the chronic diseases of aging; such as, heart disease, cancer, diabetes, high blood pressure, dementia, and joint disease like arthritis. Elevated blood sugar is associated with an elevated insulin. And, elevated blood sugar usually is associated with someone who has excessive fat, which itself sends out hormones and chemicals that are toxic to the body. It's a downward spiral.

Glycation can be normal in the body. However, excess glycation creates problems. Proteins are meant to be slippery, to slide between cells and go into cells and organs. When a glucose molecule attaches to proteins in the body, the proteins become too large and sticky to function optimally.

To Reduce Glycation

1. *Reduce Sugar Intake*

Insulin resistance and higher blood sugar increase the chance of excessive glycation. To control your blood sugar level, eat a balanced, nutritious diet, following the Glycemic Index.

One-third of Americans are diabetic. Diabetes is directly related to weight. With obesity and/or diabetes may come heart disease, high blood pressure, dementia, joint disease, cancer.

2. *Exercise to Fitness*

Exercise is superior to diet for managing your blood sugar level — but it will not work if you continue to eat in the same old way.

Exercise should be very consistent — and daily. If you are not exercising now, start by simply going on walks. Work up to one mile, then two miles. If it's winter, get out of the stale indoor air, bundle up to stay warm, and enjoy the fresher air outdoors. Or you can always use a treadmill, or stationary bike, or stair master, or elliptical machine, etc.

For more on how much exercise you really need, see "Cause of Aging 8: Insufficient Exercise."

3. *Get Optimal Nutrition*

Nutrition is the next best tool for avoiding elevated insulin. Low-glycemic foods are the surest way to lower your blood sugar level. The easiest way to identify these foods is by referring to the Glycemic Index (GI) (see appendix).

Why is the glycemic level of your foods so important? The glycemic index of foods is a scale from 0 to 100 that identifies how rapidly a carbohydrate turns into sugar (glucose) in the body.

Carbohydrates are anything that grows in the ground: fruits, vegetables, nuts, seeds, grains. Some turn into glucose quickly and have a *high* GI (>47). Some turn into glucose slowly and have a low GI (<47).

Vegetables are generally okay; except, potatoes and corn are very high glycemic. Rice, pasta, and bread are also very high and should be avoided.

Berries are very healthy; they are low glycemic and contain many good antioxidants. Fruits like apples, oranges, peaches, and pears are okay. Tropical fruits like pineapple, banana, papaya, and mango are high.

Nuts like walnuts, almonds, and cashews are good snacks. They contain one-third protein, one-third fat (healthy omega 9), and one-third carbohydrate — and they are all low glycemic.

Alcohol turns directly into sugar and should be avoided. (*Note:* Women who have one or two glasses of wine every evening quadruple their risk of breast cancer.)

If you are going to have a treat, have it with protein or fat or fiber, because these foods slow the absorption of sugar. Similarly, a whole fruit is far better than the juice, because you are also getting the fiber.

4. *Take Supplements*

The following supplements are believed to help lower and balance blood sugar. (It is important to note that supplements vary in purity and potency.)

- *Vitamin D*

- *Alpha lipoic acid* (time released)

- *Arginine* — Increases nitric oxide, which is good both for blood sugar and exercise support.

- *Curcumin* — Potent in lowering inflammation, which then lowers blood sugar level.

- *Resveratrol* — Believed to lower blood sugar and cholesterol. May assist with diabetes symptoms and weight loss. It is also thought to have neuro-protective, anti-inflammatory, and anti-viral benefits. However, it may not extend longevity, as some are saying; studies have not yet been done on mammals, the effects of long-term use are unknown, and the benefits are not yet proven.

5. *Take Nutriceuticals*

Nutriceuticals can be helpful, too. The product "Blood Sugar Support" by Vital Nutrients contains many minerals and herbals known to help control blood sugar: American Ginseng, Holy Basil, Gymnema Slyvestre, chromium, and cinnamon.

3

Free Radicals

The biological process of *oxidation* releases free radicals in the body. The clearest way to understand what this means is a statement by Ray D. Strand, M.D., author of *What Your Doctor Doesn't Know About Nutritional Medicine:* "The same process that turns a cut apple brown or rusts metal," he wrote, "is causing you to rust inside." This is why we are to take antioxidants. We don't want to be rusting inside!

Three decades ago, before many people knew about antioxidants, I went to a cutting-edge lecture on free radicals. The audience was totally comprised of medical doctors. The lecturer asked, by a show of hands, how many took antioxidants. Practically every hand went up.

Today, if one asks who is utilizing Age Management treatments, it's also mostly medical doctors who know about it and are studying the advances. Age Management medicine is preventive care. It is new, it is different, and it is totally based on the latest in science. The public is two steps behind, however, because insurance does not yet cover the cost and, in my opinion, the government is seemingly clueless and unwilling to learn about advances in age management medicine. Government programs and insurance company regulations more deny and cut back on medical care than expand into new cost-effective treatments that will enhance life and prevent disease. These treatments are more effective and less expensive.

Free radicals are normal molecules in the body, which have a dangerous affinity to binding to our blood vessel walls, cell membranes, organs, brain, DNA, and mitochondrial DNA where energy is manufactured inside our cells. These harmful bio-chemicals that the body manufactures day in and day out — all day, every day — are believed to contribute to and initiate common diseases like heart disease and cancer, the number one and number two killers of Americans. An overabundance of free radicals, over time, results in disease, dementia, loss of energy, and ill health.

Dr. Ray Strand wrote that "over 70 chronic degenerative diseases are the result of this process. Diseases like coronary artery disease, cancer, diabetes, Parkinson's, arthritis, macular degeneration, MS, lupus, among others, are the result of small oxidative changes that occur over a long period of time."

Free radicals are usually blunted by the natural processes and systems of the body. As we age, however, these protective processes can become overwhelmed and our body produces fewer *antioxidants* to fight off the free radicals.

Menopause (women) and andropause (men) are associated with increased free radical damage; because these conditions are associated with loss of hormones, and hormones are antioxidants. Over-strenuous exercise also can increase free radical production and lead to greater oxidation; the body usually can deal with this, unless there is already other disease, too much sugar, or too much fat. However, the most common production of free radicals is caused by the standard American diet (SAD).

The types of foods we eat, as well as the amount of exercise we get, affects how many and what types of free radicals our body forms. So, how do we neutralize them? The answer is antioxidants.

To Neutralize Your Free Radicals — Antioxidants

Antioxidants help the body dispose of free radicals before they have a chance to do damage. The only question is which antioxidant is best and how much is needed. There are many expensive antioxidants. The three basic antioxidants listed below suffice for many people.

- *Basic Antioxidants*
  - *Vitamin C* (2,000 mg daily) — Water soluble. Goes to the water parts of the body.

- *Vitamin E* (mixed tocopherols, and mixed tocotrienes 800 units) — Fat soluble. Goes to the fatty parts of the body.

- *Mixed carotenes* (15,000–25,000 units daily) — Part of vitamin A. Supports both vitamins C and E.

- *Additional antioxidants for specific problems* — Selenium, grape seed extract, green tea, alpha lipoic acid, acetyl-L-carnitine, curcumin, pycnogenol, and N-acetyl cysteine (NAC, turns into potent glutathione, the "master antioxidant").

- *Some minerals* have antioxidant effects; such as zinc, copper, magnesium.

- *All hormones* have an antioxidant effect.

- *Some popular antioxidants* include Acia berry, pomegranate, and other juices, which are supposedly superior (I think they are mostly superior in price, not effectiveness).

- *Arginine* can increase the release of nitric oxide, which has an antioxidant effect and is a powerful vaso-dilator.

Nitric oxide dilates blood vessels, which increases blood flow. This is very important for the heart, brain, kidney, and liver (and is also the basis of Viagra and Cialis). Nitric oxide improves cardiac function, lowers blood pressure and cholesterol, and improves exercise performance and conditioning. It allows better blood flow to all organs in the body and the brain. Through the increased blood flow, the nitric oxide provides to the body all the nutrients, water, minerals, and vitamins it requires for optimal health, and is the basis of energy production and oxygenation throughout the body. Nitric oxide sustains life!

Louis Ignarro's research on nitric oxide (nitroglycerin), reported in his book *NO More Heart Disease,* earned him the Nobel Prize in Medicine in 1997. He learned that to stimulate more nitric oxide in the body and to create optimal levels of oxygen for brain and body functions, we need 4 to 5 gms of arginine daily.

The company Xymogen took Ignarro's formula and made *NO Max ER,* available at health-food stores in capsules and powder. The Xymogene product has potentiators in it, so the arginine has a greater effect. There is no proof yet that oral arginine capsules do what arginine does in IV form; but arginine infused via an IV does stimulate the release of the human growth hormone, which is known to be very good for us (discussed in "Cause of Aging 11: Deficiency in Human Growth Hormone).

Dr. Ray Strand also wrote: "This generation must deal with more free radicals than any previous generation that has ever walked the face of the earth... The underlying problem most of us are facing is not a nutritional deficiency but, instead, the result of oxidative stress...

Because of our stressful lifestyles, polluted environment, and over-medicated society, we do need to be supplementing... You not only replenish any nutritional deficiency within six months of supplementation, but you also optimize all of the body's micronutrients."

So, to a large degree, the healthy condition of your body is something you can control. It is important to do whatever you can.

Take charge of your health habits. Stand up for your health — and be well!

4

Impaired Natural Detoxification

Detoxification is a combination of complex chemical processes that change molecules we have eaten, drunk, inhaled, or absorbed through our skin, into harmless molecules that can be dealt with, either excreted or utilized.

There are several detoxification pathways. The first thing that happens to toxins is they get converted from fat-loving (lipophilic) molecules into intermediates that are more water-soluble. This is "Phase I."

These then get "conjugated" by one of several chemical processes in "Phase II". The most common processes are sulfation (using sulfate molecules), glucurondidation (using glucuronic acid), and methylation (using methyl groups). Other important molecules are glutathione, glycine (amino acid), and taurine (amino acid).

Drugs, hormones, and other metabolites compete for the same detoxification pathways. There is abundant genetic variability and the genes control all of these hundreds of biochemical reactions. Thus, different people detoxify, or nullify, toxins at different rates and in different efficiencies. Specific chemicals in foods have specific effects on the expression and activity of these detoxification systems.

From the *Textbook of Functional Medicine* (2005), we know that onions and garlic, cruciferous vegetables, chlorophyll, terpenoids (e.g., citrus, Ginko Biloba, menthol, camphor), bioflavonoids (e.g., citrus, pine bark, grape seed, green tea), and others all act in a complex, highly beneficial manner to improve balanced detoxification capability.

One of the body's natural detoxification processes is *methylation.* Often, the natural methylation process is slowed down because of a *lack* or insufficiency of magnesium, B vitamins, and folic acid (the reason prenatal vitamins contain a lot of folic acid). It is also estimated that 40 to 50 percent of Americans have a mild genetic defect by which they cannot *methylate* well; this deficiency can be overcome by taking extra magnesium, vitamins B_6, B_{12}, and folic acid.

Methylation is a biochemical process that goes on in the body continuously. One important function is to convert the amino acid *homocysteine* into the amino acid *methionine.* Excessive homocysteine is associated with a three-fold increased risk of heart disease, osteoporosis, and/or dementia. Thus, methylation is of great importance and many people's bodies struggle to do this efficiently.

Methylation is an important part of detoxification and also properly metabolizing estrogen. Poor methylation can lead to increased amounts of toxic estrogen byproducts (metabolites), which can increase the risk of breast cancer and prostate cancer. Since up to 50 percent of people do not methylate effectively, this could be one of many causes for the enormous increase in breast cancer and prostate cancer we have been seeing since the 1990s. Supporting methylation by taking extra magnesium, vitamins B_6 and B_{12}, folic acid, trimethyl glycine, and SAMe, or other methyl donors, may help to reduce one's risk of breast cancer or prostate cancer.

It is my opinion that breast cancer and prostate cancer risk are both more highly associated with obesity, lack of exercise, alcohol consumption, poor food choices, inflammation, and the added hormones in the cattle and chicken we eat — than it is to our own body's natural hormones. Human hormones may play a role, but I believe it is minor compared to these other factors. Also, because these cancer risks are multifactorial, the subject is very difficult to study scientifically, so no one really knows for sure.

It is important to know if you are a "poor methylator" so that corrective steps can be taken to help you avoid breast cancer or prostate cancer. You can measure your homocysteine levels and vitamin B_{12} levels with a simple blood test. Specifically for breast cancer and prostate cancer, the estrogen metabolites can be measured in blood or urine to reveal whether you are at an increased cancer risk.

Your Body's Natural Detoxification Process

Detoxification enzymes exist in a healthy gastrointestinal (GI) tract, and support for healthy gut mucosa is instrumental to decreasing your toxic load (*The Textbook of Functional Medicine,* 2005). Here are simple methods to assist your body's natural detoxification process.

1. *Avoidance*

   Avoid substances that have no health value, or might have negative effects; such as, caffeine, excess sugar, tobacco, and alcohol.

2. *Inexpensive Vitamins*

   B_6, B_{12}, folic acid (some people do best with L-methyl folate). B Complex is sometimes easier to take. N-acetyl cysteine (called NAC) is also beneficial.

3. *Methylators*

   If the first two steps don't take care of the problem, methylators may be taken. Examples are: MSM, tri-methyl glycine, SAMe (be careful with SAMe, which tends to have a short shelf life).

How Can You Know If Your Body Is Toxic?

There are many symptoms of toxicity: fatigue, joint aches, lack of energy, obesity, unexplained weight gain, watery eyes, runny nose, skin rash, depression, mood swings, irritability, lack of motivation, constipation, diarrhea, heat/cold intolerance; even serious conditions like heart disease, diabetes, hypertension, possibly cancer. Plus, it can masquerade as many conditions.

How can you know if it's toxicity or something else? To differentiate toxicity from many, many possible conditions takes a knowledgeable physician. Functional Medicine doctors and Naturopaths excel in this area. Typically not a mainstream physician, because diagnosis requires thinking and testing "outside the box."

Testing depends upon clues derived by patient history and the majority of symptoms. Tests include blood, urine, stool, saliva. These tests frequently are not covered by insurance, and may be expensive.

When should you test? That is something the physician needs to decide.

To Detox Safely On Your Own

- *Eliminate* anything to which you are allergic; especially gluten, dairy, soy, egg.

- *Eliminate* alcohol, soda, sugar, artificial sweeteners, saturated fat, trans fat.

- *Reduce exposure* to toxic substances and environments.

    Common toxins include mercury, arsenic, pesticides, herbicides, lead, glue, paint, dyes. Some people are allergic to common household cleaning products, of which many contain toxins. Many substances can and are absorbed through the skin. Avoid car exhaust whenever possible. Drink filtered water. There are thousands of chemicals around us. Be aware and avoid all that you can.

- *Eat healthy foods* to support detoxification.
    - Foods in the *cruciferous family* are very good: broccoli, cauliflower, Brussel Sprouts, cabbage, kale.
    - Foods in the *allium family* are also good: onion, garlic, leeks, chives.
    - *Spices* generally are very good: cinnamon, curcumin (or turmeric, 750-1500 mg daily), rosemary, ginger, garlic, onion, sage.
    - *Flavonoids* from tea, onions, and some citrus fruits with vitamins E and C.
    - *Polyphenols* (brightly colored fruits and vegetables).
    - *Sulfur-containing foods* like eggs, plus sulfur-containing amino acids (methionine, cysteine, homocysteine, taurine).

- *Supplements* like vitamins A, B_6 and B_{12}, magnesium, folate.

- *Supplements that can provide essential ingredients for detox reactions* — I3C (indole-3-carbynol) or DIM (di-indole methane) 300 mg daily; NAC (N-acetyl cysteine) 500-600 mg, curcumin, glutamine, glycine, taurine, milk thistle, alpha lipoic acid, grape seed extract, MSM (methylsulfonylmethane), yellow dock root, Schizandra, green tea leaf.

- *Premixed combinations,* such as Metagenic's Ultra Clear, Xymogen's I5, Vital Nutrient's Detox Formula.

- *Drink lots of purified water* to flush out toxins (half your body weight in ounces).

- *Sauna* to help remove toxins (work up a sweat to flush out toxins).

- *Avoid:* smoking, high fructose corn syrup, and fasting (which exacerbates the body's deficiencies).

- *Fish oil* (3,000 mg DHA + EPA daily).

- *Magnesium citrate* (300-400 mg daily).

- *Forskolin* helps to break down fats where toxins are stored.

- *Products* like di-indole methine, or indole-3-carbinol help to metabolize estrogen.

According to *The Textbook of Functional Medicine*, most of us have between 400-800 toxic, carcinogenic, endocrine-disrupting and gene-damaging chemicals stored in our bodies, especially the fat cells. It is estimated that 25 percent of the U.S. population suffers to some extent from heavy metal poisoning, which is extremely difficult to remove from the body and may result in a severe or chronic debilitating disease. Stored toxins cause immune system deficiency. They support the growth of bacteria, viruses, yeast, and parasites; and they may foster puzzling diseases, such as chronic fatigue syndrome, fibromyalgia, multiple chemical sensitivities, chronic neurologic diseases, and many types of cancer.

Chief Editor of *The Textbook of Functional Medicine*, David Jones wrote: "There exists a 'web-like relationship' between all systems, immunologic, neurologic, gastrointestinal, circulatory, respiratory, endocrine, and detoxification . . . relationships between environment and genetic responses."

For a more extensive discussion on over-toxicity, at-risk human fetuses, a possible connection to autism, attention deficit disorder, even cancer, and how to detoxify your body, see this book's appendix, "Toxic Nation."

5

Blood Clots

As we grow older, the likelihood of our getting a blood clot (*thrombosis*) increases. This isn't good. A blood clot in the heart is called a heart attack. A blood clot in the brain is called a stroke. A blood clot that moves from one location, such as a leg, to the lung is called a pulmonary embolus. Any of these can kill.

Over the past couple of decades, U.S. labs have discovered how to measure many different clotting factors, and we can now diagnose many different minor clotting disorders.

Factor V Leiden Deficiency is a genetic deficiency that affects about 5 percent of the population, which makes a person vulnerable to getting a blood clot. More uncommon deficiences include: Anti-Thrombin III, Factor II, Protein S, Protein C, anti-phospholipid syndrome. More will be discovered. The testing for all of these is at least $500, and insurance companies are not yet paying for screening tests; they only pay when you already have a disease.

To Keep Your Blood "Thinner"

1. *Nutritional Substances*

   - Fish oils

   - Vitamin E

   - Garlic

2. *One Low-Dose Aspirin Daily*

   An aspirin daily is recommended by cardiologists. Because these over-the-counter drugs can cause stomach problems in some, low dose 81 mg is generally recommended. I have found that 200 mg of Advil (ibuprofen) daily works just as well as aspirin, if not better; although it can irritate the stomach, just like aspirin can. "Enteric coated" aspirin does not dissolve in the stomach and, therefore, does not cause stomach irritation or ulcers.

3. *Water*

   To be well-hydrated, drink water continuously throughout the day, until maybe two to four hours before bedtime. A good rule of thumb is to drink half your body weight in ounces of water daily. For example, if you weigh 140 pounds, drink 70 ounces of water daily. This also will increase your walking, because you'll be running to the bathroom more often.

4. *Move Your Body!*

Only 16 percent of people belong to athletic clubs. That's 84 percent who do not. Let's assume 10 percent work out at home. That still leaves an enormous number of people who are not exercising. Which one are you? . . . Are you *using* that club membership?

People who exercise look younger, look better, have more energy, seem happier and have better moods, have a bounce in their step, are more positive, thinner and are more flexible. They have clearer thinking, more stamina, better bone density, fewer colds, and stronger hearts. Wouldn't you like these advantages, too?

An easy way to start is to WALK. Start out by walking in the morning, or at the noon hour, or immediately after work.

Initially, you might only walk ten minutes. So, walk every darn day! Build up your stamina! Don't be a wimp!

Consistency is important. PLAN to walk *every* day. That way, if you miss one day or even two in any given week, you still WALKED five or six days.

Once this new habit is established, stretch your time to fifteen or twenty minutes. Eventually, stretch it to twenty-five or thirty minutes.

Don't let the weather stop you, either. Dress appropriately. Plan for it, so you are not too cold or too hot. All the seasons are beautiful.

When you are moving consistently, and finding joy in the exercise, you might want to add wrist bands that weigh one to two pounds. This will add some exercise to your chest, shoulders, and upper back.

If you are ready to go to a gym, great! Some gyms have become pretty inexpensive, and there's always your community recreation center. If you are self-conscious about your female body, go to a women-only club, such as Curves.

Most gyms have trainers who can teach you what to do and the best form, so you don't injure yourself. Be comfortable in taking it slowly. Most people at gyms understand that a beginner needs to go light and slow. They are very supportive, and likely will even encourage you. Also, at gyms, people tend to meet one another, so it could become a social activity!

Exercise is an essential ingredient to good health. It doesn't mean you have to run a marathon. It does mean you need to START MOVING.

If you are already an athlete or health-club member, there are many exercise theories to employ to maximize your time and health benefit. To step it up, I highly advise working with a good trainer; also you might try interval training, various machines, various forms of aerobic-fitness machines.

Don't forget flexibility! Stretching is also important. As we grow older, we tend to become markedly less flexible, especially men. It is important to have a stretching routine, daily.

For more on this topic, see "Cause of Aging 8: Insufficient Exercise."

6

Stress

Have you noticed that all of our presidents' hair turned white *while* they were serving their four to eight years? That is visible stress. We don't see what is going on *inside* the body: plaque in the blood vessels, elevated blood sugar (maybe diabetes), high blood pressure, weakened bones and muscles, affected mental cognition; and changes to the lining of the intestines, which makes absorption of food, minerals and vitamins less efficient and greatly diminished, and weakens the immune and detoxification systems.

Whatever stresses us — emotional, physical, toxin, infection, temperature too high or too low, lack of adequate sleep — causes excess cortisol to be secreted into the body. Cortisol is a stress hormone from the adrenal glands. It protects us in many ways. It regulates the immune system and is an anti-inflammatory. We cannot survive for more than one day without cortisol. The problem is when our body produces too much, which stimulates reduction in muscles, ligaments, and bones — and puts on fat!

How much cortisol in the body is too much? It's difficult to say. When we are dealing with a tremendous amount of inflammation, our body may need a tremendous amount of cortisol to deal with it.

The effort should be to lower the behaviors that promote the response of cortisol release. Such as, lower too much stress, too much sugar, hidden food allergies, over-exercise, too much fat (intake and visceral belly fat). Having said that, some cortisol lab values considered excessive are typically seen in a disease state called Cushing's Disease; and cortisol lab values considered too low are associated with another disease state called Addison's Disease.

Normally, cortisol levels start relatively high first thing in the morning. In fact, high cortisol is what wakens us every morning at about the same time. Then cortisol falls all day, until in the evening it levels off to a relatively low level. It starts climbing again during the wee hours while we are asleep. Increasing the amount and quality of sleep helps to balance your cortisol output.

To Manage Your Stress

Stress affects all of us. In days of old, stress was running from a saber-toothed tiger or a bear. It happened infrequently. Today, stress is a constant companion.

Find your stress outlets. De-stressors are activities that bring you joy, bring a smile to your face, lighten your step.

Exercise is perfect. Working out or playing a sport allows you to unwind and increases your level of fitness. You also burn off some of the stress hormones that have accumulated during the day. At the same time, the activity can be a social interaction.

If you can't bring yourself to exercise, many people relieve stress by singing, dancing, enjoying music or art, drawing, crafts, reading, going to movies, visiting with friends, taking a steam or sauna, meditating. Some people find help through classes on dealing with stress.

One calming nutritional supplement that may reduce a strong physical stress response (anxiety) is GABA (gamma amino butyric acid), which you can find in a health-food store. Progesterone also works by stimulating the GABA receptor. In addition, some people find the sublingual vitamin D to be calming, at least in promoting sleep. Some herbals, like chamomile tea, are also calming.

Sleep

Adequate and deep, restful sleep is perhaps the most important element in managing stress. The average American gets by on only five or six hours of sleep each night. However, one never really "gets by." It does catch up with you.

Americans are exhausted. With exhaustion comes despair, a poor outlook on life, a feeling of hopelessness, a lack of stamina or drive. Then along comes weight gain, high blood pressure, neurotic behavior. I am amazed at the percentage of my patients who have a sleep disturbance or an inability to fall asleep or stay asleep.

We need seven-and-a-half to eight hours of good uninterrupted sleep every night. This allows the brain to "reboot" and problem-solve (you can fix problems in your sleep, and wake with a solution in your mind). Deep sleep also gives the body's cells time to rid themselves of toxins that have built up. It allows the immune system to resupply its troops. It allows the digestive system to rebalance and resupply the cells that line the gut lumen. And it gives your heart a chance to rest at a slower pulse. All of this is what keeps you healthy, mentally and physically, and can add years to your life, good years.

So how can you improve your sleep? Try meditation or a rhythmic sound that is soothing (e.g., white noise, fan, sleep machine).

If you must, try melatonin, or time-released melatonin (two, up to 18 mg each night). You'll have to experiment with the dosage to see what works best for you. Melatonin is a hormone made in the brain, so it is natural to the body; as we age, however, our body makes less and less of it. Melatonin is also an antioxidant, so it helps to *clean* the brain. This helps to keep the brain clear and sharp — so you always know where you are, and why you came into the room.

Sometimes magnesium citrate helps with deep sleep. Magnesium is calming. It is the most utilized mineral in the body, and most of us are deficient. However, take this supplement "to tolerance," which is different for each person. Generally this works: a 200 or 300 mg tablet one nightly the first week, two nightly the second week, three the third week. Keep increasing the dose until you get diarrhea; then drop back to what you tolerated the previous week and continue that dose.

Other things people try with varying success include: herbals such as Valerian Root, or GABA, or 5HTP. Even then, sometimes sleep can be elusive. If you have "adrenal exhaustion," for example, that causes cortisol levels to be abnormal. Cortisol is supposed to be low at night. With some people, however, it is relatively high at night and that can keep you awake. To diagnose whether you have "adrenal exhaustion," and you've tried everything else, your cortisol level needs to be measured four times throughout the day: first thing in the morning, at noon, dinner time, and bedtime. This can be done as a salivary test.

If none of the above treatments work, I recommend professional help with a psychologist or psychiatrist. Sometimes, a problem with sleeping may go beyond self-treatment, and getting proper outside support may be all you need (including diagnosing if you have a sleep disorder).

Whatever you do discover that helps you go into deep, restful sleep regularly, do more of it. Make the time for it. Find that special activity that helps you unwind. It's worth it.

7

Insufficient Nutrition

The foods we eat affect our DNA. That's right. Food is not only calories.

Proper *nutrition* is almost impossible for the average American. U.S. food sources are no longer healthy. With the huge corporate farms and altered farming techniques, the nutritional value of our foods has plummeted. Genetically modified foods have become mainstream. The nutrient content also has been diminished by poor soil and an overuse of fertilizers. We are growing large fruits and vegetables, yet increasingly they are void of nutritious value.

What does this portend for our future? Nutritious foods turn on healthy genes. Empty foods turn on unhealthy genes.

Genetically modified foods (GMO), outlawed in Europe, are shown to have tremendously bad effects upon offspring. Animal studies are frightening. In animals, GMO seems responsible for genetic defects and deformity in the offspring, although it doesn't seem to affect adults. We need long-term studies on humans to know the real answers. And these studies need to be done prior to the continued use of GMO seeds.

In developing genetically modified foods, scientists added code information into the genes of plants to help protect them against pests and bacteria. The concern is that we do not know what these altered plant genes are doing to the human body; and some of the information we *do* have is not good. So, until studies have been completed, we need to outlaw GMO foods like Europe has. Unfortunately, it is probably too late; almost all of our vegetables are now GMO. For much more information, watch "The World According to Monsanto". It is shocking to realize that these foods are different than our original vegetables, and we have no choice in whether we consume them or not.

In addition, food manufacturers are making "new" foods easy and fast to prepare. However, these "foods" are full of sugar, salt, calories, trans fats, excessive and needless calories, and unhealthy signals to our DNA. They do not contain the vital nutrients, vitamins, and minerals that our body needs. Poor nutrition (e.g., fast-food industry) leads to disease and a shortened lifespan. Solid nutrition is essential for good health and longevity.

So, modern food suffers from poor soil and GMO seeds. Ideally, a fruit or vegetable would be consumed within three days of harvest, but that rarely happens. Also, it may be harvested at the wrong time;

missing the influx of vitamins, minerals, and phytonutrients (the things that protect plants from disease, bacteria, fungus, etc; also protects us) that occur during ripening. They may be damaged during shipping, or sit on a dock too long. They may sit in the grocery store for too long, or be refrigerated at the wrong temperature. In addition, we may lose much of the nutritional value by overcooking. By the time we are actually able to eat such a food, it may be very low in any nutritional value at all.

Optimal Nutrition — To Fuel Your Body

1. *Lean Protein*

Protein sources include: meats, generally from animals like cattle, buffalo (bison), deer, elk, lamb, pork; as well as fish, poultry, eggs, milk, nuts, legumes and, to some degree, seeds. A typical serving is three to four ounces. An easy measure for a single serving is the size and thickness of your palm (4 ounces). (The size of a deck of cards is equivalent to three ounces.)

Most people eat much larger portions than the body needs to function optimally. However, the body must have protein. Unlike with fats and carbohydrates, our body does not manufacture protein; and it needs it to build bone, muscle, some tissues, and to make enzymes and neurotransmitters.

I think we all realize that muscle is made from protein. Bone *also* has a protein scaffold upon which calcium is then placed to solidify the structure. We always hear that calcium is needed for bones, but protein is also needed. Neurotransmitters in the brain, like serotonin, also rely upon protein consumption.

As an aside, we all lose one pound of muscle per year if we are generally sedentary. Only 16 percent of Americans after age forty belong to a gym or recreation center, and work out. Consider where you will be at age sixty, seventy, eighty! You could be down twenty/thirty/forty pounds of muscle! This causes frailty and falls. The most common diagnosis upon admission to a nursing home is a fall.

Protein is made up of several amino acids strung together, which are the precursors to the brain's neurotransmitters. For example, tryptophan (amino acid) changes into 5-hydroxy tryptophan (5HTP). This then changes into serotonin, which is associated with mental health. Lack of serotonin is often the cause of depression. Finally, serotonin changes into melatonin, which helps us to sleep, and it is a good *brain antioxidant.*

According to Diana Schwarzbein, M.D., in her book, *The Schwarzbein Principle: The Program,* men need 13 to 23 ounces of protein daily; women need 8 to 18 ounces of protein daily. She recommends 125 grams of carbohydrates daily, and cautions that if you are diabetic or have metabolic syndrome, you need to be extremely active (exercise) and you may need 150 to 175 grams of carbohydrates daily.

Dr. Schwarzbein recommends plenty of monounsaturated and short-chain fats; and to avoid all damaged fats (trans fats, rancid fats, partially hydrogenated oils, and fully hydrogenated fats).

Fats are not the enemy, as long as they are the "good" fats. Fats are needed by our body. They are good energy sources, and they provide satiety when we eat.

Generally, eat 2 grams of carbohydrate for every 1 gram of protein (1 ounce of protein equals 7 grams of protein).

An average woman, 5'6" tall, weighing 140 pounds and moderately active, should consume 9 to 11.25 ounces of protein (63 to 78.75 grams); this equates to 126 to 157.5 grams of carbohydrates.

An average man, 6' tall, large frame, weighing 180 pounds and moderately active, should consume 11.75 to 14.50 ounces of protein (82.25 to 101.5 grams);. this equates to 164.50 to 203 grams of carbohydrates.

If you wish to know more about your personal requirements, go to Schwarzbein's excellent book where there are tables and many guidelines.

2. *Low Glycemic Carbohydrates*

We need *some* carbohydrates. However, we only need *adequate* calories to run the body's engine (often we are fighting to keep the calories lower). See the discussion above regarding the quantity of carbohydrates, the discussion on insulin and glycemic foods in the chapter "Cause of Aging 10: Insufficient Hormones," and the Glycemic Index in the appendices.

3. *Good Fat.*

We need *some* fat. Fat gives food flavor, satisfies hunger, and is essential for the brain, nerves, cell walls, and energy. We need to *increase* our consumption of good fats. Omegas 3 and 9 (polyunsaturated fatty acids) are essential for the human body.

It is trans fats and saturated fats we need to avoid. We get an overabundance of Omega 6s in the standard American diet (SAD). Excessive amounts become stored as fat and are inflammatory. So, we need to minimize Omega 6 fats, which come mainly from vegetable oils like corn oil and safflower oil, some from animal fats.

Omega 3s are found in cold-water fish and are anti-inflammatory. Omega 3s have been found to be the oil most usable by the human body. Omega 3s also come from flax seed, which has good protein and fiber — but fish oil is molecularly much closer to what our body utilizes, making it twenty times better for us than flax seed. Omega 9s come from nuts, seeds, and avocados.

I recommend Omega 3 fish oil supplements at 3,000 mg or higher daily, for both men and women. We all need them badly. We are all deficient in Omega 3s. With the standard American diet, we are way out of balance in our fat consumption.

You can get flavorless fish oils from several sources (e.g., www.nordicnaturals.com, www.vitalnutrients.net). Whole Foods and Vitamin Cottage carry Nordic Naturals regular fish oils, and Carlson's. Dr. Barry Sears, author of the *Anti-Inflammation Zone Diet* and the *Zone Diet*, sells his own highly purified oils at his website. Nutrilite (www.amway.com) has very good fish oils, called Ocean Essentials, in their Balanced Health (one needs ten capsules daily).

Why Is Omega 3 Critical for Our Health?

Our cell membranes are two-thirds comprised of Omega 3 fatty acids. Our hormonal and immune system receptor sites are intertwined with our cell membranes, too. We need healthy cell membranes for all of our body's cells to function properly and for nutrients to get where they are needed. Nutrients need to be able to flow *into* the cells; and the cells' products, like proteins and enzymes, must be able to flow *out* of the cells to go where they are needed. Our cell membranes need to be *fluid.*

Most of us are dealing daily and continuously with low grade and silent inflammation. Inflammation is a part of the immune response employed to defend us against invaders, like viruses and bacteria. An enormous body of scientific literature now links *inflammation* to chronic degenerative diseases like heart disease, vascular disease and stroke, cancer, diabetes, joint disease, dementia, and all those diseases that end in "itis" (e.g., colitis, phlebitis, arthritis).

Inflammation gets "turned on" by obesity, high-insulin levels, "bad fats" like omega 6s, hidden food allergies, and oxidation (free radicals). Omega 3s put out the fire.

Clinical Update 2010

The July issue of *Pediatrics* and the August issue of *Stroke* reported: "Omega 3 Fatty Acids Critical in Pregnancy. . . . Five year old children whose mothers received DHA versus placebo, while breastfeeding, scored higher on a test of sustained attention. In a recent animal study, researchers found that healthy omega 3 fatty acid status during pregnancy protected offspring from neonatal brain injuries."

I recommend that pregnant women take at least 1,000 mg of EPA + DHA daily. I believe that 2,000 mg is even better; you cannot get too much. This is important for fetal brain development, because two-thirds of the brain is comprised of omega 3s. The fetus is making millions of cells, and all of those cell membranes are also made up of two-thirds omega 3s. Pregnant women also need to take a minimum of 1,000 units of vitamin D_3; maybe more, depending upon their measured level of vitamin D in the blood.

4. *High Grade Vitamins and Minerals*

Many vitamins and minerals are in vegetables and fruits. We need ten servings *each* day (more than the average two or three of most Americans). A serving is equal in size to your fist. It's not a lot! A salad is a good way to mix it up, including several servings of various vegetables or fruits.

Brightly colored vegetables and fruits contain polyphenols. These are substances made by plants for their own self-defense. If you think about it, plants are at a big disadvantage compared to us. They are stationary and have to withstand everything that comes their way: insects, bacteria, drought, heat, wind. So, they developed defenses. Part of their defense is polyphenols. These are good for plants; they are also good for humans.

We get polyphenols from food, particularly the colorful vegetables; which is why we are advised to eat the colorful vegetables and fruits and to have a colorful plate of food. Other notable sources of polyphenols (which also include flavonoids) are berries, olive oil, chocolate/cocoa, walnuts, peanuts, borojo, pomegranates, popcorn, yerba mate, tea, coffee, grapes and wine, and beer. Quercetin is also a polyphenol. Although the health benefits of polyphenols are not yet proven, research indicates they are antioxidants and may reduce the risk of cardiovascular disease and cancer.

I also recommend a good multiple vitamin/mineral made from whole plant concentrates. Optimal amounts of high-grade vitamins and minerals, to prevent disease, are not cheap. Multivitamins are pretty much worth what you pay for them. There is much misinformation and false advertising associated with vitamins. A reliable website (www.consumberlab.com) is a kind of "Consumer's Report" for vitamins, minerals, and herbals. The Consumer Lab has evaluated hundreds. If you cannot find your vitamin on their site, the vitamin company either would not submit their product to testing or it didn't pass Consumer Lab's testing. The Consumer Lab's *number one multivitamin/ multimineral* listed is Nutrilite's Double X (www.Amway.com). That's the one that I take, because it is so good and contains whole food concentrates. It is full of all vitamins, and loaded with the energy-producing B vitamins. It is also full of many minerals and trace minerals, many of which are involved in producing energy. It also has many antioxidants, and some of the more rare forms like alpha lipoic acid and quercetin. In addition, it contains twenty-three fruit and vegetable phytonutrients, derived from real food sources, which is far superior to any other multivitamin.

When studying for Age Management Boards, I had to learn nutrition. As I learned about various ingredients we all need daily, I rechecked Double X along the way, and I have been continually amazed that this one vitamin contains most of what nutritionists and scientists are recommending. Double X dissolves easily in water, which is the best form for the body to utilize. It truly dissolves. It is salts that become colloidal (evenly dispersed). Double X has more phytonutrients than the next best five multivitamins combined, according to ConsumerLab.com.

Most minerals can be acquired through a varied diet of fresh foods. If we need a multiple trace-mineral supplement, it's best to get one that is analyzed for content and is bound to *citrate,* or chelated; absorption studies have exhibited acceptable and predictable absorption characteristics. You may find more information on this topic at www.WellVet.com.

5. *Probiotics*

I also recommend probiotics (the "good" bacteria). Probiotics restore and maintain the normal flora in the intestines. After living twenty to forty years or more, most humans have come across something that imbalances their normal flora: antibiotics, stress, too much of one food type (sugar in particular), toxins, illnesses (especially those that weaken the immune system, like leukemia and other cancers).

Advertisers try to sell yogurt as healthy because it has lactobacillus in it; however, the amount of bacteria is ridiculously low. It's like spitting into the ocean, trying to raise the water level.

The bacteria in probiotics are carefully chosen not to interfere with normal bowel function. They number in the billions of organisms in each capsule; the two most common are lactobacillus and bifidus. Find potent probiotics with live bacteria at your health-food store.

6. *Lots of Water!*

Whatever you weigh, divide your weight by two. That is the number of ounces of water you need to drink every day, *throughout the day.* For example, a 150-pound person needs 75 ounces of water *daily.*

A Healthy Gut

The digestive tract or "gut" has a huge role in achieving and maintaining our natural weight as well as our overall health. Diana Schwarzbein, M.D. teaches about patients who do everything asked of them and still don't lose weight and don't feel much better. Often, she later discovered that these patients were having problems associated with their gastro-intestinal tract ("gut").

The "gut" starts with the mouth, where we must chew our food adequately. Many of us eat hurriedly and don't chew well enough. This makes it difficult for the digestive system to break down food into substances that can be absorbed into the body. Proteins must be broken down into amino acids. Fats must be broken down into the building blocks of fatty acids. Complex carbohydrates must be broken down into glucose ("simple" sugar). So, first, we need to break down our food by *chewing,* so the enzymes will do their work.

The first digestive enzymes are in saliva. Then in the stomach is an incredibly high level of acid, which is essential for digesting proteins and absorbing vitamins, especially B. A lack or insufficiency of acid can set up digestive problems. As we grow older, we tend to have diminished stomach acid and B vitamins don't get absorbed, and we may become anemic ("pernicious anemia").

Even though too much acidity is often the diagnosis, frequently the real culprit is *too little* acid. When there is too little acid, the exit of the stomach (the pylorus) doesn't open completely and the stomach cannot empty easily. This initiates regurgitation. Most people turn to antacids. In fact, they need *more* acid. Antacids and protein pump inhibitors are over prescribed, in my opinion; also, now many of them are over-the-counter (OTC) and are being abused. A physician trained in Functional Medicine, or a holistic physician, can guide you in the most appropriate treatment.

In my own practice, generally I advise against using antacids and, instead, suggest using apple cider vinegar mixed in water and taken with meals. This treatment is helpful when there is, in fact, too little acid. If the vinegar is helpful, Betaine capsules (contain hydrochloric acid) taken with meals aid digestion. However, if the symptoms increase with the vinegar, then antacids are appropriate.

As food leaves the stomach, it mixes with bile from the liver and gall bladder, which aid in emulsifying fats. Next, digestive enzymes come from the pancreas to aid in protein digestion. Even the "normal flora" of the bacteria in the colon aid in digesting the food. The bowel wall is a special membrane that, if unfolded, is the size of a tennis court; it absorbs the good substances (amino acids, fatty acids, glucose, vitamins, minerals, water) and repels the bad substances (bacteria, viruses, toxins, heavy metals, pesticides, herbicides, insoluble fiber).

Most of our immune system (70%) is in the bowel, defending us from the bad substances that can make us sick. Breakdown at any level in the digestive process — inadequate chewing, poor saliva, inadequate stomach acid, inadequate bile salts, inadequate digestive enzymes, being constipated, having the normal flora affected or afflicted by antibiotics or toxins, or having a breakdown in the membrane called "Leaky Gut Syndrome" — can have an adverse outcome.

Leaky Gut Syndrome

Leaky Gut Syndrome is particularly onerous. Most people don't realize it's going on, and it can go on for years, until finally you get very sick.

Leaky Gut was not accepted as a medical condition by traditional medicine until recently. Once, it was only the realm of Functional Medicine practitioners and naturopaths.

The symptoms are similar to Irritable Bowel Syndrome (IBS). People with either diagnosis suffer from debilitating gas and gas pain, cramps, diarrhea or constipation, cravings, inflammation, and possibly malnutrition. It can affect mood and cause anxiety and/or depression. You can be overweight and malnourished at the same time.

How Do You Get a Leaky Gut?

An abnormality is created in the gut, and the cells that line the gut wall become disjointed. Normally, adjacent cells are smashed together tightly, without gaps between the cells. However, the only way anything gets from inside the intestine is to be absorbed through the cells that line the gut wall.

This requires adequate digestion of food. So, all foods must be broken down; allowing the amino acids, fatty acids, and sugars to be absorbed into the body through the cells that line the gut wall.

However — whether by viral, toxin, antibiotic, high fever, etc. — some cells separate just enough that *some* partially digested food, especially protein, "leaks between the cracks" and gets *behind* the cells that line the gut wall, where the immune system resides. This is where the "centurions" are watching what is coming through the cells and judging the material to be friend or foe. If foe (bacteria, virus, foreign protein, partially digested protein that "slipped through the crack"), the immune system mounts an attack to defend and destroy. The immune system is called to arms and becomes even more reactive. This is an *inflammatory immune response.*

The leak happens again at the next meal, then the next meal, and so on. As the "leaking" continues, the immune system becomes more and more excited and vigilant. It gets very hyped up and begins reacting to all kinds of foods — looking like food allergies.

Now, the person begins developing more and more allergies. Maybe a cough, a rash, a runny nose. Inflammation rises at an alarming rate and, with the inflammation, along comes cortisol to put out the fire.

After months of this, the immune system gets worn out and unable to respond effectively. You start getting frequent colds and infections. The adrenal glands get worn out from producing incredible amounts of cortisol, and you may get *adrenal exhaustion.*

Now you feel absolutely horrible because you don't have enough cortisol to do all the many things it normally does daily. Incredible fatigue sets in and you are very easily exhausted. You don't feel like doing *anything.* You get *joint aches,* which is sometimes confused with arthritis or fibromyalgia. Because your cortisol levels have been chronically so high, you *gain weight.* Even exercise, at this time, only makes matters worse, not better; because exercise requires healing post exercise, and healing requires cortisol.

So, exercise requires cortisol, and the person with adrenal exhaustion doesn't have enough, or any. The little cortisol that might have been used for something else is now used by the exercise event. No cortisol means feeling exhausted, achy, shaky, flakey. Plus, oxidation is now free to exist far too much; this further creates damage to the body, making it more vulnerable to disease or illness, because the immune system is also exhausted and is "down."

This is a downward spiral that feeds upon itself. The best way out is to heal the Leaky Gut! To do that, your doctor must know about Leaky Gut (few do). The doctor must know which tests to run to make the diagnosis, and must know how to reverse the Leaky Gut process and promote optimal health. To date, few doctors have learned this.

You can find a trained and experienced physician at www.functionalmedicine.org. This could be an M.D. (medical doctor), D.O. (osteopath), D.C. (chiropractor), or N.D. (naturopath). Like all things in life, there are great and poor levels of care provided by any discipline. My bias is that while medical doctors have a great deal of integrity and knowledge, many resist change and may not be up on the latest research findings. There are many exceptions; in studying "alternative medicine," I have learned that each medical discipline has some extremely brilliant people. Even so, it is buyer beware.

The tests to diagnose Leaky Gut include a "Complete Digestive Stool Analysis," which might require a four-point cortisol test. Also, there might be stool cultures and permeability tests.

Once the diagnosis is made, treatment varies depending upon the individual's situation. It likely will include digestive enzymes, probiotics; gut calming agents like glutamine, aloe or fish oil; special shakes for calming, healing, treatment. You might even need antibiotics, but that can do more harm than good, so caution is advised. You likely will be put upon a "rotation diet."

Optimal Health Plan

Dr. Diana Schwarzbein's GI Panel (complete digestive stool analysis), from her book *The Schwarzbein Principle: The Program: Losing Weight the Healthy Way,* an easy, five-step, no-nonsense approach, is helpful to figuring out what is going on with your intestinal tract. She defines five key areas to keep your body whole and in balance:

- *Nutrition*

  Besides what you eat, vitamin and mineral supplements.

- *Stress Management*

  For adults, uninterrupted sleep for seven to eight hours *every* night, helps to cope with everyday life stress.

- *Exercise*

  Thirty to sixty minutes of exercise every day is essential for emotional equilibrium and mental clarity, as well as longevity. How much exercise depends on your current fitness level and meeting your nutritional needs. (Remember that exercising to excess actually creates cortisol-producing fat.)

- *Detoxing*

  Stopping and cleansing sugar from the body yields the most remarkable results; as does removing alcohol, nicotine, caffeine. The results come from healing and down-regulating the negative responses to these drugs and chemicals, using up energy, and getting out the chemicals that decrease brain function and muscle function, etc.

- ***Hormonal Balance***

    Estrogen and progesterone for women. Testosterone, DHEA, thyroid, and human growth hormone for both men and women.

Testing your gastro-intestinal health, using the Schwarzbein GI panel, requires three different stool samples, plus saliva samples. It checks: the most abundant immunoglobulin in the gut, SIgA; the four most common food allergies (wheat, milk, egg, soy); digestive enzyme levels; cell damage related to Leaky Gut; and levels of bacteria and bacterial overgrowth, yeast contamination, and parasites. Once the diagnosis is made, comprehensive and specific treatments can yield slow but astonishing results.

Healthy intestines mean a healthy body. Getting your gut healthy and functioning normally again can turn everything around in how you feel. Optimal nutrition then will feed your entire body; providing abundant energy, vitality, and wellness.

8

Insufficient Exercise

E *xercise* is the kingpin of abundant health. It is the *number one way* to combat elevated blood sugar levels. Exercise reduces the risk of cancer and heart disease (the two top causes of death in the U.S.) by 50 percent, including breast cancer. It helps to control weight and obesity. It enhances the circulation of blood and nutrients to all organs in the body, especially the brain.

In his two newest books about the effects of exercise on the brain, *A User's Guide to the Brain* and *Spark: The Revolutionary New Science of Exercise and the Brain,* John Ratey, M.D. wrote that "aerobic activity can transform not only the brain, but the mind as well" and also affects "learning in children."

In these two books on "exercise and its effect on mood, cognition, anxiety, attention, addictions, and aging," Ratey added that exercise even has "a huge impact" on disorders such as "aggression, autism, and ADHD" and "helps kids to regulate their moods and balance their emotions; stimulates their cognitive abilities; and helps them feel motivated. . . . Exercise activates the brain" by spawning a "release of brain chemicals known as neurotransmitters, and improves the flow of blood and oxygen to the brain." As a result, one feels "brighter and more alert." For people over the age of fifty, exercise is shown to "push back cognitive decline by 10 to 15 years" and women "derive more benefits . . . especially after menopause."

What Form of Exercise Is Best?

The one that you will do!

Humans were designed to move. We need to move and stretch *every* day. Stretching daily prevents us from becoming unable to move. Stretching is the key to maintaining mobility and avoiding injury.

Only 20-25 percent of the population exercises routinely. Yet fit individuals suffer fewer injuries and less illness. They have more energy and less depression. They look and feel younger.

Exercise is critical to vitality, energy, weight control, general health, and longevity. Elevating the heart rate for thirty to forty-five minutes increases fitness and endurance.

The goal is to maintain some muscle strength and flexibility. Without that, one might fall; which is the most common precipitating factor that leads to admission into a nursing home. Women, in particular, become too frail without exercise.

Without exercise, we lose one pound of muscle *every* year. Consider this going on for thirty or forty years! To avoid becoming a weak and frail little old lady or man, we need to maintain strength, flexibility, and vigor for all of our days.

As we grow older, we need to do more resistance type of exercises and less prolonged strenuous exercise; for example, *weight lifting* with recovery periods between sets. *Pilates* is extraordinary for building "core strength." *Yoga* is terrific for stretching and strengthening; *hot yoga* is performed in a room heated 103-105 degrees (personally I think that's overboard, good sweating I suppose).

If you are sedentary — Simply start moving. *Walking* is a good way to start. Go for a five-to-ten minute walk daily at lunch time. Gradually increase the time and effort or pace. Work up to walking one to two miles every day. *Note:* Consistency is most important.

Once this is mastered, add some wrist weights of one to two pounds. Walking exercises and strengthens the calves, the quadriceps and hamstring thigh muscles, the gluteus muscles (butt), and the abdominal muscles; but it doesn't do much for the upper body. Adding the wrist weights gives some resistance for the chest, upper back, shoulders, and arms.

Exercise also may involve different types of workouts. Choose your favorite. Some people like the "great outdoors" and enjoy hunting, walking, hiking in the wilderness. Some like fishing and fly fishing; again, hiking into remote areas. Hiking, climbing, backpacking, skiing, snowboarding, and ice skating are healthy activities.

Some people prefer fun activities like aerobic dancing, Zumba dancing, NEA aerobics, or weight aerobics.

Some people prefer to swim. With water aerobics, you can have a very physical workout in the water. Running in water is an excellent way to get in shape; water is twelve times more resistant than air (so movement through the water is challenging). Water is also buoyant, so it is easier on joints, especially knees and hips.

There are many aerobic fitness machines: stationary bikes, spinning classes, group biking, elliptical machines, stair stepper machines, recumbent bikes, and treadmills. Start slow. Gradually work into more demanding activities and longer times on the machines. *Spinning* is riding a stationary bicycle with varying resistance; typically an instructor leads the ride and you increase or decrease the resistance at various times to simulate riding up and down hills. The *elliptical machine* is like a treadmill with a motion like running; your foot moves in an elliptical pattern.

If you are fit — Engage in recreational training or sports; such as tennis, golf (walking, not riding in a cart), hand ball, racquet ball, softball, baseball, basketball, soccer. Any activity that involves running.

If you want more fitness — Get into resistance training with either weights or machines, and integrate different techniques. You can work on individual muscles and strengthen weak areas; people like to improve biceps, triceps, deltoids, latissimus dorsi, pectoralis, and trapezius muscles. The following four motions are fundamental for the upper body: (1) lift weights above your head and shoulders (military presses); (2) the opposite motion, like a chin-up, pull from above downward; (3) lie on a bench and push the weights upward (bench press, strengthens chest muscles); (4) pull something toward you in a rowing motion (strengthens upper back). If you are a novice, I recommend getting advice from a trainer.

If you are very athletic — You might like interval training, high intensity weight training, rock climbing, even marathons and triathlons (too much for most people).

Surely, out of all of these options, you can find at least one regular activity that is fun for you as well as challenging?

Why, again, should you exercise? Just to live longer? No. To live well! To slow and minimize the effects of biological aging!

The Fundamental Benefits of Daily Exercise

- Normalizes blood sugar level.

- Lowers LDL (unhealthy) cholesterol.

- Improves HDL (healthy) cholesterol.

- Improves focus. Mind is clear.

- Normalizes weight! (As long as you also follow a reasonable eating program.)

- Stimulates lymph flow through the body, carrying away debris and toxins. (The lymph glands are the body's detox channels for draining what you want to wash out of the body. Improving lymph flow improves draining the swamp.)

- Increases stamina and endurance! You are fit!

- You have a wonderful feeling of well-being.

  For more on this topic, see "Cause of Aging 5: Blood Clots."

Your Optimal Body Weight

Two-thirds of Americans are overweight by at least 20 pounds; a third of Americans are obese, generally 30 pounds over the ideal weight for their height. Our children also are more obese than ever in recorded history, and increasingly more so year by year. Exercise and nutrition are the solution.

Let's break it down. Let's help you reach your optimal weight. How?

You need optimal nutrition, optimal exercise, and a good level of fitness. You need stress management, the greatest of which is adequate sleep. You need total hormonal balance. When all of these factors are aligned, your weight normalizes and the body can heal whatever needs healing. When the body is operating at its prime, you are biologically *young!*

A healthy *metabolism* maximizes an *optimal* weight and body composition. If you attempt to lose weight with a damaged metabolism, you can further damage your metabolism. Even with a healthy metabolism, "fad dieting" (e.g., diet pills) usually damages the metabolism. Such "dieting" raises the cortisol levels too high. So, rather than "diet," *optimize* your weight.

To Reach Your Optimal Weight and Slow the Aging Process

- Strive for great nutrition (whole foods, avoid sugars)

- Utilize supplements as needed

- Exercise daily

- Practice stress management

- Plan adequate sleep (adults, 7-8 hours every night)

- Achieve total hormonal replenishment and balance (replenish low levels of hormones to *optimal* levels).

My mother always told me, "Eat well, do your work, and stay out of trouble." Every day, we can be active and vital, for however many days God gives us. We can bob along happy and healthy, until one day we just don't wake up!

87

9

Shortening of DNA Telomeres

Aging is very much controlled by our *telomeres*. These are the end caps on each DNA strand. They are involved in maintaining genetic stability and in regulating cellular life span. Telomeres are involved in normal aging, and in several diseases like cancer, heart disease, and others.

Our telomeres shorten at different rates under different healthy or unhealthy circumstances (healthy food choices vs. unhealthy food choices, exercise vs. no exercise, hormones vs. insufficient hormones). Telomeres dictate the life span of our cells; therefore, the life span of an organ. So, telomere length is very important to our *biological* age. Measurement of telomere length tells us our biological age.

Telomeres control the number of times a cell divides before it dies. Every time a cell divides in the body, our DNA is replicated and a small piece of that DNA's telomere is consumed in the process. Because of this loss of part of a telomere, division by division, eventually that cell's DNA runs out of telomeres and cannot divide again. After approximately eighty cell divisions, that telomere is totally used up and the cell dies.

We don't actually know much yet about extending the length of telomeres. There is a medication advertised to stimulate telomerase, which lengthens telomeres; however, it is speculated that increasing telomerase might increase cancer risk. This company states that their product "TA-65" raises the level of telomerase; however, most of our cells do not have the ability to *make* telomerase. The company also states that "TA-65" makes one look and feel younger, relieving aches and pains, improving vision, increasing strength, energy and stamina. The fear that scientists have of making telomerase, however, is the potential of inviting in cancer; because if the old ragged cells don't die, as they are supposed to do, the old worn out cells might become cancerous. There is promising research; however, I don't believe we know enough yet to be promoting or taking a telomerase-enhancing product. Currently, we don't have the safety data. In fact, I believe it is quite risky. No good clinical studies, published in first line big name journals, have been completed at the time of this writing.

Interestingly, some cells do have telomerase, the enzyme that actually *regenerates* the telomeres. Some white blood cells, germ cells, and stem cells have this telomerase. This guarantees that we won't run out of blood or sperm (so the species will live on). And it is important that we continue to generate more stem cells.

Cancer cells have the ability to maintain and lengthen *their* telomeres because they have telomerase, essentially conferring immortality upon the cancer cells. So, there is a tremendous quantity of basic research on telomeres, how they function, what protein signaling is going on, and what that might mean in terms of being able to control the process. Not only for their anti-aging aspects, but to figure out why cancers become immortalized yet normal cells do not.

In summary, telomeres have everything to do with aging. *We do know* that people who are fit and exercising, are not overweight, have better nutrition, and are supplementing hormones, have longer telomeres. Longer telomeres is associated with better health.

Here are some supplements that are proposed as enhancing telomere length:

Copper, folate, glutathione, magnesium, selenium, zinc, B vitamins, Vitamin C, Vitamin D, Vitamin E.

Things you can do to enhance telomere length:

Reduce oxidative stress (oxidation and free radicals)
- o Diet low in sugar, avoiding fast food, soda, high fructose corn syrup
- o Minimize emotional stress
- o Lower physiological stress like infection
- o Increase antioxidants

o Lower inflammation

Reduce cardiovascular risk factors

o Low blood pressure

o Minimize carotid intimal thickness

o Lower homocysteine

o Lower C Reactive Protein

o Raise HDL

o Lower LDL

Increase Exercise

o At least 30 minutes daily

o Suggests a 10 year younger biological age!

Maintain healthy weight

o Low body fat (>16% men, >22% women)

o Decreasing visceral fat

Lower insulin resistance and metabolic syndrome

o Shortened telomeres are independent predictors of diabetic complications

How long are your telomeres?

10

Insufficient Hormones

Men and Women

We grow old because we lose our hormones. All of us. Women *and* men.

When it comes to slowing and minimizing aging, total hormonal replenishment is the most vital treatment. Hormones are fundamental to everything about us: our physical body's functions, how we feel, how well our brain works, if our emotions are even.

In short, for both men and women, the human body runs on a messenger system called the hormonal system and the nervous system (neurotransmitters). Every cell, every organ, every function in the human body is dictated by these messengers.

This chapter overviews why hormones are so vital to all of us. The next two chapters focus on replenishing deficiencies in the human growth hormone and the brain's neurotransmitters. Then, most significantly, "The Women's Guide" and "The Men's Manual" detail exactly which hormones are needed for the female and male bodies to function optimally.

When Does Aging Begin?

Disease does not happen overnight. Most of us are pretty healthy until about age thirty-five or forty. Then things begin to change. At forty-five, fifty, or fifty-five, we go to the doctor and learn that we have diabetes, or high blood pressure, or America's #1 killer of both men and women, heart disease. *High blood pressure* can damage organs, and it does lead to injury of the lining of arteries; as cholesterol tries to heal the damage, the blood vessels get plaque, making them less elastic and less able to absorb the pulse waves of the beating heart. Whatever we've got, it's been in the making for a decade or more.

The body makes itself over again and again. Hormones control and regulate many systems in the body. They are essential for our survival. They tell our body's cells what to do, when to do it, and how much.

As we acquire more and more birthdays, our hormones plummet. Disease begins to set in and obsolescence processes are going on; such as, inflammation, oxidation, glycation, poor methylation, poor detoxification, increased blood clotting. Our body is in disarray and our immune system doesn't function properly. Our *brain* doesn't function well; we are forgetful, irritable, and we don't reason as well as we once did. Our *heart* is exposed to more plaque, arrhythmias, and smaller caliber vessels that have less elasticity. Our *bones* become osteoporotic, brittle, and fragile. Our *skin* loses elasticity, causing it to wrinkle; the *vagina* becomes dry and uncomfortable (*intercourse* becomes painful in women as the vagina loses elasticity). *Colon* cancer goes up. *Bladder* capacity shrinks and it becomes leaky.

Without hormones, the body goes into chaos. To live healthfully and to our full potential, we *all* must have the hormones estrogen, progesterone, testosterone, and DHEA. *All of us. Men as well as women.* Without *these* hormones, we can certainly live; however, we cannot reach our full potential and not without nagging debilitating diseases. None of us can live without hormones; and not much more than one day without the major hormones insulin and cortisol.

Menopause affects most women's hormonal levels to a significant degree. Men, however, are totally unaware of what's hitting them; it comes over them slowly, stealing their energy, their competitive spirit, their passion for life, their libido. It's like watching your children grow but you don't really see it.

A good part of the body's obsolescence process is in the way our hormones alter their functions as we age. We lose 1 to 2 percent of our hormones *every* year! That's 14 to 20 percent *every* decade! The only hormone that does not decline is cortisol, and it is not our friend — it makes us fat!

Hormones are molecules usually produced in a gland. They distribute throughout the body via the blood vessels; they target tissues and bind to receptors in cell membranes. Hormones direct cellular function. They signal the production of proteins for structure, fats for membranes, and chemicals to heal, repair, and restore cellular integrity. Hormones are the life-giving signals that keep the body functioning in harmony.

So, when our hormones decline, we have more health trouble (disease). Perhaps the immune system isn't as good as it used to be and we aren't able to fight off cancer. Maybe our repair mechanisms are faulty or running very slowly and we recover poorly after a workout or an injury. Maybe we have more difficulty utilizing glucose for energy and we have an abundance of glucose left in the blood vessels; this means a higher blood sugar level that, at some point, will become "sugar diabetes."

Depending on the type of hormone, the signal may have a different effect. Depending on the type of cell, the signal may be interpreted differently. However, the hormones tell the cells to *do* something; like make a protein, an enzyme, or an antibody; or let something *into* the cell, such as glucose (insulin does that).

Our body is made up of fifty to seventy *trillion* cells. Some cells are sloughing off, some are being made to replace those at a remarkable rate. Each cell membrane is covered with over one thousand receptor sites; and each cell membrane is comprised of two-thirds omega 3s, as in fish oil. These receptor sites are for specific hormones; there is a specific receptor for insulin, estrogen, testosterone, thyroid, and so forth.

For example, steroid hormones are sterols; think of it as a protein. The steroid hormones are made in a gland: thyroid gland, ovary, testicle, adrenal, pituitary. From the gland, they enter the blood stream and circulate throughout the body via the blood vessels. They eventually make their way to a cell, bind with the receptor on that cell, and send a signal inside the cell, often directly to the DNA. Receptors are specific for specific hormones; they live in cell membranes and are very dynamic. Other hormones, like immune system hormones, are not sterols and are not made in a gland.

Why do we lose our hormones? No one knows for sure. I believe it has a lot to do with our lack of good nutrition, lack of exercise, toxic environment, viruses, inflammation, oxidation, glycation, and poor methylation.

To balance the body's hormones, women need to pay attention to their estrogen, progesterone, testosterone, DHEA, thyroid, and vitamin D. In menopause, women can be deficient in all of these; balancing them is very important to a woman's total health, because hormones work together synergistically. For more on the critical functions of women's hormones, see "The Women's Guide" later in this book.

As men age, they need to replenish their levels of testosterone and DHEA, and usually vitamin D. More rarely, men might need thyroid supplement. For more on the essential hormones in the male body, see "The Men's Manual" later in this book.

Bio-identical hormones are the safest supplementation for both women and men. The most effective form is absorbed through a transdermal patch or cream or troche (lozenge); the correct individualized dose achieves the optimal level of hormones.[3]

So, maintaining hormonal balance is essential to the quality of life and a properly functioning body. Hormones are critical for good physical, mental, and emotional health.

Pituitary Gland Directs Our Hormones

Many hormonal systems operate like a thermostat. A thermostat measures the amount of heat in the air. When it gets cool enough, the thermostat sends a signal to the furnace to "make more heat." The furnace fires up and makes heat. When the air becomes warm enough, the signal to the furnace turns off, then the furnace turns off and stops making heat. The cycle goes on and on.

Similarly, our *pituitary gland,* which sits centrally at the base of the brain, reads how much hormone is running around in our body. The "thermostat" analogy applies to the steroid hormones estrogen, progesterone, testosterone, DHEA, and thyroid. In the same way that the pituitary reads the thyroid level, it also measures how much estrogen is in the blood stream. When the amount of estrogen gets too low, the pituitary sends it's hormone messenger FSH (follicle

---

[3] The concept of "biologically identical" hormones was popularized by Suzanne Somers in her book, *The Sexy Years,* in which she adroitly points out the structural differences between human hormones and those derived from animals and plants.

stimulating hormone) via the blood stream to the ovaries, which stimulates the follicles. It is the follicles in the ovaries that produce estrogen and are the source of the majority of estrogen in women. When the pituitary reads the increased level of estrogen in the blood, it stops sending FSH and shuts down the signal.

The broader idea is that we must maintain a fairly strict balance so that all our hormones operate synergistically together; because hormonal deficiency (e.g., menopause, andropause, hypothyroidism) results in various physiological changes, below the optimum level of our vigorous youth. Hormones that need to be regularly reevaluated and rebalanced, for optimal well-being in both women and men, are estrogen, progesterone, thyroid, testosterone, DHEA, growth hormone, insulin, and cortisol.

If we can't see well, we wear eyeglasses or contacts. If we have diabetes, we take insulin to correct our elevated blood sugar levels. If we have appendicitis, we have surgery to correct the body's imbalance. If we have an infection, we take antibiotics. Why not correct a hormonal deficiency and — get your body back!

The Three Hormones That Are Key to Life

Without cortisol, adrenaline, and insulin, we would die in one or two days. When our level of any of these hormones is chronically elevated, or there is a chronic degenerative disease (e.g., Type 2 Diabetes), we have a damaged metabolism that needs help. When these hormones respond normally to stimuli, we have a healthy metabolism — which keeps us feeling and looking great!

Cortisol

Both cortisol and adrenaline come from the adrenal glands, and are released with stress. When we experience "adrenal burnout," we have very low amounts of these two hormones.

Cortisol is released more with *chronic* stress. Stress can be emotional but also from physical causes; such as infection, heat or cold, parasites, lack of food, food allergy, toxic overload. Chronic stress eventually will result in adrenal burnout.

Most Americans live in a world of constant stress and have elevated cortisol levels. This tears down the body, taking protein from the muscles, ligaments, and bone. Plus, cortisol stores fat, especially around the middle (apple shape).

Cortisol's major function is to moderate the inflammatory response. It is frequently called the "stress hormone" because it calms the inflammation response and initiates healing.

The level of cortisol in the bloodstream varies normally. It starts high in the morning, waking us up at the same time every day. It falls all day long, reaching its nadir around bedtime. Then the level starts building in the wee hours of the morning, peaking and waking us up again for another day.

Adrenaline

Both cortisol and adrenaline turn on sugar production and raise our insulin level. As this happens, they also shut down any burning of fat, pushing the body into fat storage. Adrenaline uses up not only protein but also carbohydrates and fat, robbing the body of what it needs for routine functioning.

Adrenaline is the *immediate* response to stress. It mobilizes us to fight or flee. It increases our heart rate and blood pressure, dilates our pupils for better vision, and heightens our awareness. Adrenaline puts our brain into high drive, so we can think quickly. It mobilizes our blood sugar to enhance our energy, and gives us the fuel to carry out a task quickly. Frequently, people end up with trembling, sweating, and/or heart racing to some degree, depending upon the stimulus. Typically, this response is short-lived, maybe two to three minutes.

A second stimulus on top of that, such as a fright, may elicit a reduced response because the body may or may not have enough stores of energy left to respond sufficiently. The end result is exhaustion, until recovery occurs.

When acutely stressed, adrenaline causes the heart to race; you feel shaky or may have an inner trembling. Over the long haul, this may result in adrenal burnout. People with *adrenal burnout* are miserable and have difficulty functioning in even daily routines. Recovery takes months and can be a slow process. However, recovery is possible. Changing lifestyle is the most difficult part of this process.

The solution to stressors in the old days was to kill that saber-toothed tiger. Nowadays, stress is usually more subtle, and removing the stress from our lives is often impractical, if not impossible. So, our best solution today is to employ any number of stress-reduction techniques. There are numerous classes. In some situations, a person might benefit from psychological therapy. For others, the answer is going to the gym and physically working stress out of the body.

A simple way to learn if you have "adrenal burnout" or "adrenal dysfunction" is a *saliva test* that measures your levels of cortisol throughout the day. You collect the saliva sample when you first arise, again at noon, again at dinner time, and again at bedtime. The test is about $200; insurance typically doesn't cover it. When I run this test, I reserve it for people who are dramatically fatigued or having a great difficulty sleeping.

Many doctors are afraid to try to correct an adrenal deficiency, because they don't understand the dose. There are those of us who are knowledgeable and proficient at utilizing low doses of cortisol when necessary. Stopping the symptoms is accomplished by correcting either the cause of the burnout or the hormonal deficiency itself.

Insulin

Insulin is a hormone that increases in the blood stream when we eat, especially refined sugars and simple carbohydrates. Insulin takes the glucose out of the blood stream and transports it into the body's cells to be used as energy (or stored as fat). Insulin also transports amino acids into the body's cells to build protein, enzymes, and neurotransmitters; or to convert them into glucose, or fat, depending on what the body needs.

The human body operates like a hybrid car that runs on both gasoline and electricity. When the car uses up its electricity, it turns to gasoline. *When the body uses up its sugar, it turns to burning fat.*

However, if the insulin in the body is elevated, the option to burn fat is not available, even though fat may be abundant. Controlling sugar and insulin, keeping their levels low by utilizing the Glycemic Index (see appendix), allows your body to shift from sugar-burning to fat-burning — exactly what you want.

Average Americans chronically have relatively high insulin levels. When carbohydrates are high, insulin is released. High insulin levels stimulate both cortisol release and inflammation; these are the core cause of most chronic degenerative diseases: heart disease, cancer, hypertension, stroke, diabetes, arthritis. Cortisol breaks down muscle, ligament, and bone — *and* puts on fat. As long as your insulin is elevated, you cannot burn fat. When elevated from ingesting high-glycemic carbohydrates (refined sugars, processed foods, simple carbs), you *will not* burn fat. Thus, it is very important to decrease your sugar intake!

To lose weight, you *must* lower your sugar and high carbohydrates intake. This shifts your metabolism into *burning* fat! Then you can lie around for eight hours every night and still burn fat!

Fat is not the enemy. Sugar and *high*-glycemic carbohydrates are the enemy. To lose weight and maintain weight, for good health and a balanced metabolism, eat by the *Glycemic Index* — six days a week.

On the seventh day, indulge a *little* in *one* thing you enjoy. Then cycle back to the low-glycemic eating plan. The point is to eliminate "poor food choices" most of the time, and enjoy them only at *selected* times.

Glycemic Index Foods

With 30 to 40 percent of men and women diabetic and 10 to 20 percent hypoglycemic, 70 percent overweight and a third of those obese or morbidly obese, following the Glycemic Index for how and what to eat has become a critical health issue.

The Glycemic Index (see appendix) helps us to choose healthy kinds of foods. The glycemic rating between 0 and 100 indicates how rapidly a specific food raises the blood sugar and insulin. This is analogous to a speed limit on a highway — the lower the number, the lower the blood sugar, and the safer our vehicle, our body. For a healthy metabolism, choose foods with a glycemic index under 47.

As stated in the chapter "Cause of Aging 7: Insufficient Nutrition," carbohydrates are anything that grows from the ground: fruits, vegetables, grains, nuts, seeds. Not all carbs affect blood sugar in the same way. High-glycemic foods stimulate a significant rise in blood sugar, followed by a significant rise in insulin. The problem is that insulin returns to normal more slowly than sugar; so when your blood sugar has restabilized, your insulin is still elevated. You don't want that.

Normally, after sugar is consumed, the body turns to its other fuel, fat. However, when the insulin is elevated, the body *cannot* access the fat as fuel, so it sends a signal — a craving. Typically, we reach for the wrong "food" (e.g., bagel, donut, brownie, candy).

This is one of the major reasons children in America are obese. They consume 50 percent of their calories as high-glycemic carbohydrates. They are not burning off the carbs. Instead, they are storing it as fat.

Changing this behavior is a key component to weight loss and weight control. When we eat low-glycemic foods, our insulin doesn't spike as high, and it gets down to normal as the blood sugar level returns to normal. Then the body can access and burn the fat as fuel.

So, you can be a fat burner or a fat storer, depending upon your dietary choices. This is enormously important to understand. Controlling your carbohydrates intake is the key to *sustained* weight loss and maintaining your *optimal* weight.

There are fad diets, low-fat diets, HCG diets (dangerous), and all kinds of ways to try to trick yourself into weight loss. If you are serious about weight control, learn the Glycemic Index and follow it for the rest of your life. It works. I know. I lost thirty-five pounds by doing this!

The Three Hormones That Are Key to Good Health

Thyroid, vitamin D, and DHEA are "minor hormones" that are critical to good health and longevity.

Thyroid

The thyroid gland produces an essential hormone in both men and women. It controls the rate at which the body's cells work, which is the metabolic rate (metabolism). One statistic says 5 percent of the population is hypothyroid; however, there is disagreement on this. As many as 20 percent of menopausal women *are* deficient in the thyroid hormone; and 2-5 percent of men over the age of forty. It is safe to say that women are hypothyroid far more often than men.

Thyroid deficiency — hypothyroidism — is associated with weight gain, slower thinking, sluggishness, sleepiness, fatigue, lack of energy, constipation, dry skin, and depression.

The pituitary gland in the brain reads the thyroid level in the blood stream. If the thyroid hormone is too low, the pituitary sends a hormone messenger called TSH (thyroid stimulating hormone) via the blood stream to the thyroid gland. In response to the TSH, the thyroid produces more hormone, solving the problem of too little thyroid hormone. Once the level of thyroid hormone raises to a sufficient level, the TSH shuts off and the thyroid gland shuts down until the next time TSH comes to stimulate further production.

Many doctors measure only the TSH in a thyroid screening test, which is often insufficient and even inaccurate. The thyroid gland makes T4 (thyroxine, a pro-hormone), which converts in the body into T3 (triiodothyronine), which is what the body uses. However, about 10 percent of people have trouble converting T4 into T3. Therefore, the levels of *Free* T3 (FT3) and *Free* T4 (FT4) *also* need to be tested.

In the bloodstream, thyroid hormone is bound to a protein thyroid-binding globulin (TBG). A small percentage (1%-2%) is not bound. Thus, it is "free." It is the free fraction of the thyroid hormone that is the active and *usable* portion of the thyroid hormone, which also needs to be tested.

The TSH should be between 0.5 and 2.0; even though labs erroneously quantify the "normal level" up to 4.5. *Free* T3 should be between 3.0 and 4.4. *Free* T4 should be between 1.0 and 1.8. Some holistic doctors, including myself, recommend Armour Thyroid medication to rebalance the T3 and T4, because this ground-up pig thyroid closely resembles what the human body makes and includes *both* the T3 and T4 forms of thyroid hormone. However, because some people react to the "foreign" pig protein, some doctors (including Dr. Diana Schwarzbein, endocrinologist) prescribe Synthroid. The problem is that this bioidentical thyroid is mostly only T4; for those whose bodies do not convert on their own, T3 can be added as the bioidentical thyroid Cytomel.

Another potential measure of thyroid function is Reverse T3 (RT3), which is a mirror image of the T3 thyroid hormone. RT3 can occupy a thyroid receptor, but it doesn't turn it on. So, RT3 blocks T3 action by taking up a receptor but doing nothing. In this way, RT3 is a brake on the thyroid system. Sometimes, if people receive too large a thyroid dose, their RT3 elevates. Cortisol, the stress hormone, shuts down the conversion of T4 to T3, and increases the conversion to RT3; this can make you slightly hypothyroid, but serves to calm you down. RT3 also may be elevated by gluten intolerance/Celiac, low B_{12}, and/or low Ferritin (iron storage hormone).

A marker of autoimmune thyroid disease is thyroid peroxidase (TPO), so this antibody titer can be used to assess disease activity in patients. Autoimmune Hashimoto's thyroiditis is a fairly common disease, and usually results in hypothyroidism as the thyroid "burns out" from inflammation. Thus, TPO is a marker of Hashimoto's thyroiditis.

Anti-thyroid antibodies are directed against the thyroid gland, or thyroid hormones; for example, thyroxine (T4) and triiodothyronine (T3). These antibodies, usually associated with inflammation of the thyroid gland, affect its function. Antithyroglobulin and antimicrosomal antibodies are types of antithyroid antibodies. Testing for these antibodies in the blood is useful in diagnosing some thyroid disorders; such as, Hashimoto thyroiditis (autoimmune thyroid disease), Graves disease (overactivity of the thyroid), hypothyroidism (underactivity of the thyroid), thyroid cancer, lupus, rheumatoid arthritis, autoimmune hemolytic anemia, and Sjogren's Syndrome.

When the thyroid hormone level is correct, people do feel better. They have a more appropriate weight and more energy. Find a doctor who looks beyond only the TSH levels. Ideally, someone in Functional Medicine. You'll need an M.D. or D.O., because they are the only doctors with the legal ability to prescribe.

Iodine

To make adequate amounts of the thyroid hormone, the body needs an adequate amount of iodine, a mineral that is an ingredient in thyroid hormone production.

Many people are low on iodine. If our body doesn't have enough iodine, or amino acid tyrosine, our thyroid hormone production may be inhibited, creating the hypothyroid state.

It is estimated that 90 percent of Americans are iodine deficient, because we have no dietary source for iodine other than iodized salt, and that is not enough. The fact is we don't get much iodine in the standard American diet. Iodine was added to bread until the 1960s. Then bread makers switched to bromine instead, which is similar to iodine; however, it competes with iodine for the same binding sites in the body, and it does not turn on the binding site as iodine does. Iodine *is* in standard table salt, but many people try to avoid too much salt because of blood pressure. Also, if you are using sea salt — it does not contain iodine (iodide).

Lack of iodine also may be the cause of fibrocystic breast disease. So, iodine is good for both thyroid and breast health.

How Can You Know If You Are Getting Enough Iodine?

There are no symptoms to know if you are iodine deficient.

A urine test through a lab can check your iodine level. First, you take 50 mg of iodine. Then you collect all of your urine for twenty-four hours, and a lab measures your level of iodine in the urine. This is somewhat difficult to accomplish.

Here is a simple and inexpensive test you can do at home. Pick up tincture of iodine at any grocery or drugstore. Use a cotton ball or gauze to rub *some* on your abdomen, two to three inches wide. Keep the iodine away from good clothing, because it stains.

Put the iodine tincture on in the morning. Check the area about every hour and see how long it takes to fade. If the stain on your skin lasts more than twenty-four hours, you have adequate iodine stores in your body. If it goes away sooner, you likely need an iodine supplement. If it goes away in two to four hours, you are very iodine deficient and you do need an iodine supplementation (Idoral tablets, available OTC in compounding pharmacies). After taking this iodine supplement (Idoral) four to six weeks, repeat this skin test. When you go more than twenty-four hours, you can stop taking the Idoral.

There is a great debate regarding iodine. Some medical practitioners believe that iodine is necessary, since there are three or four iodine atoms on each thyroid hormone of T3 and T4; the iodine atoms reside on two tyrosine molecules that are hooked together to make the thyroid hormone. However, in some people, iodine seems to depress the thyroid production. So, some physicians recommend taking the amino acid tyrosine. Personally, I haven't seen this to be very helpful, in most cases. So, I prefer to test thyroid production as well as the iodine level, to assure a proper balance in both in the individual.

DHEA

DHEA is the most abundant hormone in the body, and the majority of it is made in the adrenal glands. It is a *precursor* to estrogen, progesterone, testosterone, and cortisol. However, taking a DHEA supplement will not raise the levels of these hormones significantly.

When women's ovarian hormones estrogen, progesterone, and testosterone fall with menopause, most often the adrenal hormone DHEA also falls. Likewise, as men lose testosterone in andropause, their DHEA levels typically drop.

Women who have a higher level of DHEA, such as through supplementation, may get a very small boost in their natural testosterone level, because a small amount of DHEA converts into testosterone in women. In men, however, especially weight lifters and body builders, it does *not* convert into testosterone.

Benefits of DHEA Supplementation

- #1 Benefit: Boosts immune system (helps to fight colds, flu, and other viruses).

    Cancer fact: Viruses cause cancer. So, DHEA should help to fight cancer.

    Some medical researchers believe that cancers are formed in the body almost every day, but that our immune system destroys them. If this is true, we want our immune system functioning at full force all the time.

    There is an enormous amount of research regarding HPV (Human Papilloma Virus) and cancer of the cervix. We now have a vaccine to partially immunize young women against this Human Papilloma Virus, which causes cervical cancer.

- Protects the brain and breasts.
- Increases feeling of well-being (called the "feel good hormone").
- Enhances sexual response and libido.
- Helps to maintain lean body mass (muscle) so you don't grow frail.

- Increases weight loss.

    In a study of a group of older people who were given DHEA, their average weight loss was 14 percent!

Typically, take DHEA in pill form, although it is available in a cream and lozenge. The average female needs 10 mg; the average male 25 mg. Average includes mostly menopausal women and andropausal men, or people with one or more illnesses. Each individual responds differently. To assure that you neither overdose nor underdose, you need a knowledgeable physician to properly manage your optimal level.

A potential negative side effect of DHEA is that some women experience an increase in oily skin or acne. The same thing can happen to men.

If this happens, stopping the supplementation returns the skin to normal. In these cases, many women can switch to 7-keto DHEA and receive the benefits without the acne side-effect. The typical dose for women is 25 mg daily; for men, 25-50 mg.

When lab tests are completed and reports printed, the lab typically prints out what they call "normal." However, what you want is *optimal.* I have found the printed reports with the "normal" range to be far below optimal levels needed for feeling your best and being your best. The correct interpretation of the data is crucial for a superior health outcome.

Vitamin D₃

Want to feel better — physically *and* mentally? An obvious and common symptom of vitamin D deficiency is general all-over aches and pains in the bones, joints and muscles, along with muscle weakness. Depression also may be a factor.

Vitamin D deficiency affects the entire body: the brain, immune system, mood, temperament, muscles, bones, organs, cells, insulin production in the pancreas, metabolism, and hormonal balance. Even though Vitamin D is truly classified as a vitamin, it has many hormonal-like actions, which are discussed here. Possibly 2,000 genes are regulated by the *hormone* we call vitamin D; 6 percent of human genes are directly or indirectly affected. This deficiency is also a factor in obesity. Over eight hundred published studies in the nutritional literature state that a vitamin D level tested in the range of 60 to 80 will cut in half one's risk of *all* cancers. So, a vitamin D deficiency is a quite significant issue.

New research is being reported frequently, revealing more and more benefits of vitamin D. In *The Vitamin D Solution,* Michael F. Holick, M.D., Ph.D., a pioneer in vitamin D research, describes how obese people are lacking sufficient vitamin D. He discusses studies that show how higher doses of vitamin D significantly affect recovery in breast, prostate, and colon cancer; in some cases, improving survival rates by 39 to 48 percent. This new research even has inspired a new understanding of the "genesis" of cancer in the body and has provided bold new theories in cancer research.

Most Americans are deficient in the hormone vitamin D. However, the body doesn't make D on its own. The most efficient way to get it is through sunshine, which is converted by the skin into vitamin D. To get adequate D from the sun, we need to expose 75 percent of our skin at midday (skimpy swimsuit) when the sun is most intense, for at least twenty minutes; that amount of time is not harmful to the skin regarding skin cancer. Dr. Michael Holick reminds us that sensible sun exposure occurs in the spring, summer, and fall. He points out that our skin is best stimulated by the sun to produce vitamin D between 10 a.m. and 3 p.m.

However, because we avoid the sun or wear sunscreen or sunblock to protect our skin from cancer and sun damage, we are not getting enough sun exposure for converting sunlight into vitamin D. Also, when you feel lousy, you just want to be a couch potato. You don't want to go out in the sunshine.

Fortunately, there are other ways to boost vitamin D in the body! Foods that naturally contain small amounts of vitamin D include fortified dairy products (whole milk, butter, cheese), salmon, mushrooms, and fortified orange juice. However, these sources are typically insufficient, so we really do need daily sunshine as well as supplementation to meet the body's health needs.

Recent studies show that we need a much higher dose than the 400 units approved by the FDA (even the recent increase to 600 units). Both are significantly insufficient! I have found that most people need 2,000 to 4,000 or even 6,000 units daily.

We don't need to be overly concerned about overdose of vitamin D; it is fat soluble, meaning it isn't secreted through the kidneys. With 95 percent of Americans tested as deficient in vitamin D (test levels below 60), the existing concern about possible overdose seems overstated. No one truly knows what level is toxic in the blood stream; however, it is believed to be around 250. To be safe, I regularly measure the patient's vitamin D level in the blood stream. So anyone taking vitamin D should be monitored by their physician with lab tests. The optimal level is 60-80; some holistic practitioners recommend up to 100.

The good news is vitamin D is inexpensive, even in high doses. You easily can buy it at any health-food store in capsules or drops. I also have found that one or two sublingual drops under the tongue at bedtime helps many people sleep better.

Benefits of Higher Doses of Vitamin D₃

- Burns calories (more metabolically active, fat-cell metabolism).

- Decreases risk of cancer by 50 percent.

- Decreases insulin resistance, so the insulin works better and the blood sugar level is lower. (One study reported by Michael F. Holick, M.D. showed a risk reduction of 33% in Type 2 Diabetes.)

- Is a powerful anti-inflammatory.

  Inflammation is the greatest risk to our long-term health. So supplementing vitamin D is one of the most important considerations to avoid the chronic degenerative diseases of aging.

- Helps immune system (so less frequent colds and flu).

  In *Life Extension* magazine (Sept. 2010), Dr. Holick reported that adequate D in children may help to protect them against viral and bacterial infections; also evidence from studies suggests that Type I Diabetes may be caused by "an initial viral infection." Dr. Holick has listed levels of vitamin D for children at 400-1000 units; for teenagers and adults at least 1,500-2,000 units daily.

- Better mood, less depression (stimulates production of serotonin).

- Helps female ovulation.

- Increases sperm count in young men.

- Helps to protect against sunburn — while absorbing into the skin!

- Aids in absorption of calcium (helps bone density and muscle strength).

   One concern about vitamin D is that it does aid in calcium absorption. This is good, except we don't want calcium going to our arteries, only to our bones. Vitamin K_2 helps to direct calcium preferentially to the bones; thus, I recommend taking 100 mcg of K_2 with vitamin D_3.

It is always recommended to have your vitamin D level checked, which can be done by a simple blood test at any lab. Look for a level between 60 and 80; actually, below 100 is okay. If your level is below 60, you *do* need supplementation. For example, one woman's test at a local hospital lab came back at 28; by standard medical practice, this was considered only modestly low, because the traditional range for "normal" starts at 32. I must say, however, that according to recent studies, that is very insufficient for optimal health, and supplementation is essential.

To test your vitamin D level, Functional Medicine doctors measure a 25-OH vitamin D_3. If that stays low and doesn't respond to treatment, they then look at the 1, 25-OH vitamin D_3. (Some uninformed doctors look only at a 1, 25 D_2 or the 1, 25-OH D_3.)

Why Take D₃ and Not Just D₂?

Vitamin D_2 is the generally accepted and prescribed vitamin D. However, the body needs *both* of these forms. D_2 is often prescribed in 1.25 mg pill form to be taken once a week (50,000 units), and it may have side-effects. I don't understand why one would take this massive amount once a week. I think the body would do better getting a moderate dose every day. That is why I recommend, and utilize myself, 2,000 to 6,000 units of natural vitamin D_3; which is four times more potent than D_2, more is absorbed, and it is well-tolerated.

Both D_2 and D_3 are available over-the-counter. Most people need 2,000 to 6,000 units daily, depending on their personal vitamin D level in the blood stream. The recommended daily allowance (RDA) recently raised from 400 to 600 units is *far* below the latest recommendations of experts in the field. I recommend periodically to retest your vitamin D level to see how you are doing (every four to six months). Also, keep in mind all your sources of vitamin D (e.g., a single supplement of perhaps 2,000 units, the multivitamin you take, the calcium with vitamin D that you take).

In closure, think sunshine (not sunburn). Combine fifteen to twenty minutes daily of sunshine with foods and supplements. For this brief exposure to the sun, there is no need for sunscreen.

Add vitamin D_3 supplement to the sunshine and food because aging decreases the skin's ability to make vitamin D from the sun. We need all of these important resources in order to live a sunshine happy life!

11

Deficiency in Human Growth Hormone

Abetter name for this is "healing hormone." The human growth
hormone is as close as we get to the fountain of youth. Its
effects are nothing short of marvelous!

Today, doctors and healthcare professionals worldwide believe
there is direct correlation between the aging process and the gradual
decline of the human growth hormone (HGH) production in both
women and men. The general loss of energy, endurance, and other
conditions associated with aging may be a result of ever-decreasing
human growth hormone levels in the body. With replacement of HGH,
people lose weight and feel more energetic. They avoid colds and flu
better. Physical repair is more rapid. Workouts are done with more
power and agility, and there is a better maintenance of lean body mass.

Arguably the most important hormone in the body, HGH is
produced by the pituitary gland in the brain. Daily growth hormone
secretion peaks around puberty and begins declining by age twenty-

one. In our teenage "growth" years, the pituitary secretes human growth hormone at 100 percent capacity. Once we pass these growth years, the pituitary slowly reduces production by 12 to 15 percent every *ten* years. By age thirty, most people start noticing an acceleration in aging. By middle age, the production of HGH may be only 50 percent of the levels we enjoyed as a teenager. By age sixty, low growth hormone is fully evident. Even most adults >60 have total 24-hour GH secretion rates indistinguishable from hypopituitary patients with organic lesions in the pituitary gland. Aging adults not receiving hormone replacement therapy, DHEA, and thyroid frequently report fatigue, lethargy, decreased strength, and decreased exercise tolerance. Several recent epidemiologic studies indicate an increased risk of cardiovascular morbidity and mortality in this untreated patient population.

Deficiency of HGH consists of a greatly decreased quality of life, apathy, low energy, decreased muscle strength and aerobic capacity, and an atherogenic lipid profile (cholesterol, triglycerides, HDL, LDL) that makes the body very prone to atherosclerosis, heart disease, and stroke. Other alterations in the body's composition include: decreased bone mineral density, increased visceral adipose tissue (fat inside the abdominal cavity, associated with heart disease, diabetes, stroke), and increased sarcopenia (fat but starving, weight appears normal despite a high percentage of body fat).

Progressive pituitary hormone deficiency is characteristic of aging. The first hormonal system affected is the hypothalamic growth hormone, IGF-1 (insulin-like growth factor) axis. Since 1995, a large body of clinical evidence has identified Adult Growth Hormone Deficiency (AGHD) as an important cause of aging-associated hypopituitary syndrome, and has demonstrated that growth hormone therapy is effective in ameliorating *all* related symptoms. For example, growth hormone therapy has been shown to: decrease fat mass, increase lean body mass, increase bone mineral density, reduce both LDL and total cholesterol, reduce carotid-artery intimal media thickness, increase the number and function of endothelial progenitor cells (repair vascular walls), increase exercise tolerance, and dramatically improve overall quality of life.

The human growth hormone supplementation has been shown to restore muscle mass, decrease body fat, reduce wrinkles, restore lost hair and hair color, increase sexual function and energy, improve cholesterol, enhance vision and memory, normalize blood pressure, increase cardiac output and stamina, improve immune functions, and restore size of liver, pancreas, heart, and other organs.

The Fifteen Powerful Benefits of HGH Replacement

1. *Lose 14% Weight and Body Fat*

Thousands of doctors and healthcare professionals consider human growth hormone (HGH) supplementation to be one of the most effective methods of reducing body fat and controlling weight. In numerous clinical trials, the loss of deep abdominal fat was pronounced. This visceral fat is extremely hard to lose and is often associated with an increased risk of heart attack.

2. *Build 7% Muscle, Lean Body, and Strength*

Studies at the University of New Mexico indicated that young people already in good shape gained an average of three pounds of muscle and lost 1.5 percent of their body fat in six weeks. Their overall ratio of muscle to fat improved 25 percent on average!

3. *Increase Energy, Endurance, and Stamina*

The first benefits you notice after starting human growth hormone are increased energy, endurance, and stamina. It usually takes three to five weeks for all of the receptor sites to become saturated. This is a gradual process, so there is no instant gratification. However, once your HGH level reaches a certain threshold (varies person to person, based on gender and age), you feel a noticeable increase in energy and endurance. This is the tip-off that the process is working!

It is this increased energy and endurance that can bring improved levels of sports and exercise performance. A youthful level of HGH does not increase your skill level, but the resultant increase in energy and endurance enables you to work longer and harder to develop the skills of your chosen sport or physical fitness routine. In a well-known study by Thierry Hertoghe, M.D., in adults receiving human growth hormone injections, fatigue decreased or disappeared in 86.8 percent of participants.

4. *Restore and Enhance Brain Power*

Human growth hormone helps to clear brain fog. Just as our brain functioned more clearly in youth, HGH helps to restore sharp, quick brain functions and memory. Plasticity involves the functional interplay between the three major cell types: neurons, astrocytes, and oligodendrocytes. Neuro-protective effects shown in experimental models of Central Nervous System (CNS) injury increases progenitor cell proliferation, new neurons, oligodendrocytes and blood vessels in the memory center (hypocampus).

5. *Restore Youthful Skin Elasticity, Diminish Wrinkles*

As we age, our skin becomes thinner and loses its firm texture and elasticity. In a world-renowned study by Dr. Daniel Rudman, after increasing their HGH levels, elderly men had an increase of skin thickness of 7.1 percent on average. In a self-evaluation of 202 people taking HGH for six months, two-thirds reported improvement in skin texture, skin thickness, and skin elasticity. Of this group, 61 percent observed fewer wrinkles and 38 percent reported healthier hair. Patients usually started noticing changes within a few weeks of treatment. Fine lines appeared to vanish; deeper wrinkles receded and facial fat decreased, so that puffs of fat under the eyes evaporated and the facial muscles that lift and hold the skin became stronger. Another result was the elimination of cellulite.

HGH increases the synthesis of new proteins that lie underneath the skin structure. In animal experiments, HGH increased the strength and collagen content of the skin; collagen and elastin are the underlying foundation of the epidermis. HGH restored the bounciness that is characteristic of young skin, so that the skin bounced back more readily upon testing, became better toned, and sagged less.

6. *Maintain Optimum Immune System*

At puberty, our immune system functions at its peak. Today, many doctors recognize that by helping the body increase HGH to a youthful level, it goes a long way to maintaining a healthy immune system as well. Studies by Keith Kelly, M.D. and others have shown that by replenishing our level of HGH, our immune system activities all increase and intensify; including the manufacture of new antibodies, production of T-cells and Interleukin 2, proliferation and activity of white blood cells, stimulation of macrophages (pac-man like scavenger cells in the white blood cell line), increased maturation of neutrophils (main white blood cell), increased erythropoiesis (making red blood cells), and production of new red blood cells. A healthy immune system is, perhaps, the most important benefit of HGH supplementation.

7. *Repair and Maintain the Body*

The primary function of human growth hormone is the growth, repair, and maintenance of cells, organs, and body parts. Interest in the use of HGH to improve the quality of life in aging adults stems from research reporting that HGH exerts neuro-protective and neuro-stimulating effects that bolster cognition and memory in an aging brain. Studies of both men and women have shown that higher IGF-1 at midlife is associated with significantly better late-life cognition. (HGH acts partially by increasing a protein in the liver called IGF-1.)

8. *Achieve Healthy Cholesterol Levels*

Increasing the level of HGH can help to maintain cholesterol levels in individuals already within the normal range.

9. *Regulate the Blood Pressure*

Maintaining a youthful level of HGH improves cardiac and lung functions, two functions that help to maintain a healthy blood pressure. Studies by Daniel Rudman, M.D. and others have shown that increasing the HGH level reduces diastolic blood pressure by 10 percent without changing the systolic pressure (not intended to prevent or treat hypertension).

10. *Regulate Cardiac and Pulmonary Functions*

Recent studies also suggest that increasing one's human growth hormone level helps to increase cardiac function. The associated increases in energy and endurance also may lead to improvements in pulmonary function.

11. *Maintain Healthy Bones*

Raising HGH to a youthful level also can help to maintain a healthy bone mass. Many women, pre, post, and menopausal, are having much success with HGH supplementation. Also, a youthful level of HGH often goes side by side with raised levels of osteocalcin (a hormone that helps to build bone) and two types of collagen (key factors in maintaining overall health).

12. *Improve Deep, Restful Sleep*

Many studies support the fact that replenishing HGH to a youth level promotes a deeper, more restful sleep. Remember how well you slept when you were young? You *can* get back those nights when you could sleep through the loudest of thunderstorms.

13. *Enhance Mood*

Human growth hormone may just be one of the most powerful, natural antidepressants available. There is ample evidence that increasing one's HGH level helps to elevate mood and lower stress and anxiety. A higher HGH level increases the levels of neurotransmitter B-endorphine and lower dopamine. Other studies suggest that an elevated level of HGH improves one's self-esteem and, overall, a positive outlook.

14. *Restore Libido and Sexual Function*

Another study by Daniel Rudman, M.D. has shown that older men after six months of HGH injections significantly enhanced their sexual performance. Sexual rejuvenation is one of the most commonly reported benefits of an increased HGH level. It appears that as we grow older and our growth hormone level decreases, our libido and sexual functions decrease on parallel tracks. This finding has prompted many researchers to claim that increasing HGH may be one of the most powerful ways to restore youthful libido and sexual function.

15. *Restore Total Hormonal Balance*

Human growth hormone supplementation also can elevate the hormone levels in women who are pre, post, and menopausal. Menopausal total hormonal replacement can be done safely and effectively by using bioidentical hormones, balancing the estrogen and progesterone, and using the appropriate dose for each individual. HGH supplementation is both safe and effective as it relates to the symptoms commonly associated with menopause.

How To Take Human Growth Hormone

Only by subcutaneous injection. Pills, nasal sprays, and lozenges don't work; double-blinded controlled studies have shown these to be of no use. HGH is a large molecule, larger than insulin. No one yet has been able to find a way to give insulin other than by subcutaneous injection. HGH has the same problem. Avoid false advertising regarding other forms of HGH. It will waste your money and health.

Can You Take Human Growth Hormone Supplementation in Combination with Other Treatments?

Absolutely! In my practice, I measure for "optimal levels" with all the hormones: HGH, estrogen, progesterone, testosterone, DHEA, and thyroid.

How Can You Know the Right Balance for Similar Symptoms and Similar Benefits?

The levels are measured with blood tests. I find that symptoms can be misleading, so I listen to the symptoms as well as observe lab test results.

What Are the Risks of Human Growth Hormone Supplementation?

Two symptoms occur rarely: transient swelling, transient joint pain. If these symptoms do occur, you simply can reduce your dose for a few days until the symptoms go away. Then gradually increase the dose until you return to the previous dose; then that dose will be tolerated.

Seventy-five recent journal articles support the safety of HGH. Since 2007, over thirty studies, reported in major peer-reviewed journals, have supported a *lack* of cancer risk associated with HGH replacement. Despite what you might hear, or what some out-of-date doctors think, according to the numerous recent studies there is *no* increased risk of cancer from taking human growth hormone.

What Is the Cost of Human Growth Hormone?

It is expensive. What really good thing isn't? The cost for the average dose of HGH is around $500 to $600 monthly. Some insurances cover it, but many don't. How an insurance company can dictate patient care I still don't understand. How the government can dictate what a patient can or cannot have is a mystery to me. The FDA has made new rules governing the diagnosis of Growth Hormone Deficiency. While there are literally hundreds of peer-reviewed studies reported in medical journals, discussing the safety and value of HGH treatment, the FDA is single-handedly attempting to make it too difficult for anyone to "qualify" for treatment. In my opinion, the FDA is over-regulating a valuable hormone.

The effects of HGH on humans have been studied for over forty years, which has revealed that the body produces 15 percent less HGH each successive decade. HGH stimulates virtually all the various systems in the body. It increases the metabolism, helps to break down fat, builds proteins, and creates lean muscle. You reasonably can reverse ten to twenty years of age decline with one year of continual therapy. No other substance known to medical science has been shown to deter and reverse continually the process of aging.

12

Deficiency in Brain Neurotransmitters

Beginning early in life, the brain stimulates specific glands that stimulate the release of hormones, thereby controlling the hormone levels in the blood stream. These hormones go throughout the body to control the specific functions of cells and organs. These same hormones then come back to the brain and affect the brain's functions.

Bioidentical hormone therapy alters the body and the brain's chemical processes to restore strength and health in an aging body. This is critically important for both menopause (female hormonal depletion) and andropause (male hormonal depletion).

Hormone therapy also significantly improves *neurotransmitter* deficiencies and conditions affecting memory, concentration, and cognition; mood disorders, fatigue, and insomnia; even obesity, osteoporosis, libido and sexual function.

Although *neurotransmitters* are molecules that function in the brain — they are manufactured mostly in the gastrointestinal (GI) tract. So, the production of neurotransmitters is directly affected by amino acids derived from our foods and supplements.

Protein is the most important nutrient to brain chemistry; and it is comprised of a string of amino acids, which are the precursors to the neurotransmitters and are essential, even critical, to our brain's function.

The Four Major Neurotransmitters for Calming and Brain Power

For Calming and Promoting Sleep: Combine the recommendations below for serotonin and GABA, which put the brain into relaxation mode. Also, to increase calmness and help themselves sleep, some people take B vitamins and/or the amino acids leucine, isoleucine, and valine.

For Maximum Brain Power and Speed: Combine the recommendations below for dopamine and acetylcholine, which stimulate the brain.

Serotonin

A deficiency in serotonin is commonly associated with depression. An insufficiency of this brain neurotransmitter affects many behaviors and body functions, including mood.

- *Serotonin:*
  - Helps to reboot the brain every morning so we begin with a fresh start.

- Controls cravings.

- Affects the ability to rest, regenerate, and find serenity.

- Helps to promote sleep, by converting into melatonin in the body.

- Is a good brain antioxidant, by converting into melatonin.

- Is associated with pleasure, sensing, feelings, and harmony.

- *Food sources:* Turkey, chicken, pork, cottage cheese.

- *Production is aided by:* Vitamin B$_6$, omega 3 fish oil, St John's Wort.

- *Derived mainly from:* Tryptophan (5-hydroxy tryptophan, 5HTP).

GABA (gamma-aminobutyric acid)

GABA is naturally calming and is the major inhibitory neurotransmitter of the nervous system.

- *GABA helps with:* Stability, sociability, concern for others, consistency, memory, and language.

- *Food sources:* Eggs, complex carbohydrates, organ meats, whole grains, vegetables, nuts, legumes, cantaloupe, oranges, and reishi mushrooms.

- *Production is aided by:* Inositol (related to phosphotidylcholine), B vitamins, and the amino acids leucine, isoleucine, and valine.

- *Derived mainly from:* Amino acid glutamine.

Dopamine

Dopamine is closely associated with norepinephrine and epinephrine, which are involved in energetic demands and thinking.

- *Dopamine helps with:* Energy and motivation.

- *Food source:* Turkey.

- *Production is aided by:* Chromium, rhodiola, thiamine, methionine, phosphotidylserine, and B complex. Restoring depletion is aided by hormones and vitamins; the supplements Beta-Phenylethylamine, N-acetyl-L-Tyrosine, and L-Taurine; and the nutrient cofactors vitamins B_6, B_{12}, and folinic acid.

- *Derived mainly from:* Amino acid *tyrosine;* secondly from the amino acid phenylalanine (converts into tyrosine).

Acetylcholine

Acetylcholine is mainly associated with memory.

- *Acetylcholine helps with:* Thinking and brain speed.

- *Food sources:* Eggs, antioxidant vegetables, and fruits like tomatoes and blueberries.

- *Production is aided by:* Manganese, lipoic acid, huperzine-A, fish oil, and DHA; as well as choline, phosphotidylcholine, N-acetyl-cysteine (NAC), and L-carnitine.

- *Derived mainly from:* Amino acids phosphatidylserine and acetyl-L-carnitine.

Neurotransmitters is a new field. Much still needs to be discovered. Recently, labs have determined how to measure neurotransmitters in urine; they have proven a correlation to blood-level results. However, currently, it is nearly impossible to determine if the tests can measure brain health.

Nonetheless, knowing a patient's neurotransmitter levels does make it easier to identify and treat a deficiency. To date, using supplements has met with variable success.

Studies in rats have shown that a lack of sufficient *estrogen* decreases dopamine release and increases noradrenaline release; so, a lack of sufficient estrogen relates both to decreased calmness and increased anxiety. By contrast, these effects are reversed when estrogen levels are restored, increasing calmness and the feeling of well-being — which is what many patients experience with restoring their hormonal balance. (Technically, estrogen up-regulates the alpha-

1-adrenergic receptors or excitatory effect, and down-regulates the beta-adrenergic receptor activity or inhibitory effect.)

Likewise, a lack of sufficient *progesterone* significantly reduces allopregnanolone (a metabolite of progesterone). This is important because allopregnanolone, as well as DHEA (dehydroepiandrosterone), is a brain-produced neurosteroid that exerts regulatory actions on brain cells. Significantly, allopregnanolone stimulates the GABA receptor that modulates stress, mood, and behavior; thereby, reducing anxiety and increasing sedation.

In addition, bioidentical progesterone is neuroprotective, meaning it protects the brain against trauma, physical and chemical. It also helps to put a protective myelin sheath around the nerves, and it protects vessel linings (vascular endothelium). Whereas, the fake progesterone (progestin, Provera) does none of this.

These numerous distinctions between bioidentical and chemically produced progesterone and estrogen are important implications for using bioidentical hormone replacement therapy during menopause and the aging process, to protect against neurodegenerative diseases.

Also, we can alter our brain transmitters through healthy food choices. It takes several weeks (4-12), but it can be accomplished. (See chapter "Cause of Aging **7**: Insufficient Nutrition.")

Exciting news! A new medical device to determine our "brain age" will hopefully be available in 2012 late 2011 or early 2012. This is a true advance in medical care. For the first time, we will be able to identify who has dementia, and predict who will and who will not develop progressive dementia, also called Alzheimer's Disease. This groundbreaking new device, made by WAVi in Boulder, Colorado, looks something like a bicycle helmet. Nineteen electrodes are imbedded in the helmet, which read the patient's brain waves and create an EEG. Based on thousands of EEG studies, the individual EEG is then read by a computer and compared to *normal;* any abnormalities are compared to patterns of diseases like dementia, Alzheimer's, anxiety, depression, and the like. This diagnostic test will be inexpensive and done at your doctor's office in only about twenty minutes, which is incredible; currently, the only other test that comes close to this is a $3,000 functional MRI, and that requires a trip to the hospital or a lab. I will post on my website www.AgeManagementMD.com all news regarding this amazing new medical tool in understanding brain cognition and identifying brain disorders.

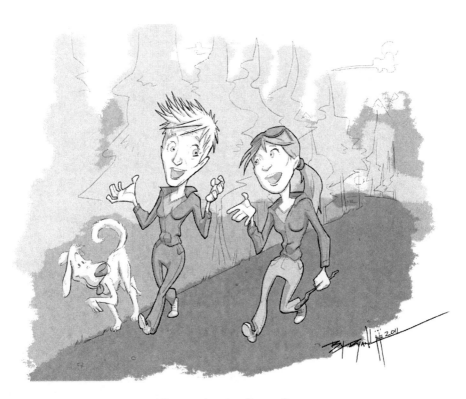

Illustration by Ryan Lee

The Women's Guide

Restoring Your Vigor, Harmony, Balance!

"It took me five years to find Dr. Lee. He changed my life. In September 2004, I had a hysterectomy, including ovaries. It turned out to be a fibroid tumor and not the cancer it was thought to be.

1. I started to have severe prickly hot flashes, then I got extremely cold from the sweat on my body. I dressed in layers summer and winter, night and day, sleeping and awake. I could no longer wear wool. I could no longer wear makeup, because it ran down my face and into my eyes due to the hot flashes. I was miserable.

2. I had to quit my job of thirty years, because I couldn't function. I couldn't think. I couldn't remember. I was tired and irritable and not myself anymore. I just thought, when you reach sixty you start to get old and die.

3. I couldn't sleep even with sleeping pills. I couldn't remember when I'd had a good night's sleep. I went from hot to cold all night long. I also urinated eight to ten times a night. I wet the bed numerous times and my doctor said I was incontinent and gave me pharmaceutical pills to control a spastic kidney. I also had nervous legs (they continued to kick when I was in bed and trying to go to sleep), so they also gave me pills for the nervous leg syndrome.

4. I couldn't remember anything. When I walked into a room, I didn't know why I was there. My brain didn't work anymore. I thought I was dying and that no one knew what was wrong. I was fading away day by day and year by year.

5. My body was drying out and shriveling up. My eyes were so dry that I tore my right one and developed eyeritis and had to put steroids in both eyes four times a day for over a year, or I would get head-throbbing headaches in my eyes.

6. I quit Kaiser in October 2009, because I was no longer in business or eligible since I had quit work. I felt I needed better medical care. I didn't find it, and believe me I looked. I just went from one doctor to the next. It got so that when I went in for an appointment, I would give the doctor a paper with all that was wrong with me, and my health history, so I wouldn't miss anything.

7. Around August 2009, I started to itch and, when I scratched, it would welt and bleed. The itch started on my back, but eventually moved to my head. Sometimes it was under my breasts or on my tummy in the form of a rash. I thought I was allergic to something, so I quit wearing nail polish, had my fake nails taken off, changed shampoo, changed detergent, etc. Finally, I went to a dermatologist and was given steroid shampoo for my head and steroid

cream for my body. It didn't help and, also on the container, it clearly said to quit using it if I noticed my skin thinning. I was told that I had Ciboria. I also went to an allergist and they found nothing; they thought it was dry skin.

8. At the same time, I noticed lumps on my arms as big as a piece of double bubble gum. I went to the same dermatologist, and he removed five in March 2010. I had so many lumps on my arms and legs that there was no way to get them all removed; I was so embarrassed that I only wore long-sleeved shirts in the heat of summer.

9. By the summer of 2010 when I would hot flash, my head and face would be soaked. I felt steam as if coming off my head. I was getting worse. I stayed in bed most of that summer. I was always tired, and I caught everything and anything that was in the air.

10. My legs hurt when I got up during the night or first thing in the morning. I walked bent over.

11. I was tired all the time. No energy. Never in a good mood.

12. I have no sex drive whatsoever.

13. I was so depressed. I was dying, and I was suicidal. I cried all the time.

14. Most days, I just stayed in bed. Well, while in bed, I watched *Larry King Live* and listened to an interview with Suzanne Somers and thought, *That's me.* That was August 2010. I went right out and bought her *Breakthrough* book and read every page. Thank you, Suzanne. Finding a doctor was not easy. I went to four before I found Dr Lee. One doctor fired me from his practice, because he had tried everything to fix me and nothing worked. When I asked him to do hormone testing (after Suzanne's book) and asked if he ever administered bioidentical hormones, he would not answer. After asking three times, I went for a second opinion; he got angry and fired me from his practice. This was one doctor before Dr. Lee, and this doctor gave me other medication but would not give me bioidentical hormones and I was not getting better.

15. A friend said to please call Dr. Lee ... so I made an appointment with Dr. Lee, expecting the same idiocy I had found with the other doctors. I wanted to live a normal life, so I had to keep trying to find a doctor who knew how to fix me.

"I walked into Dr Lee's office.

1. I saw him one on one, and he didn't rush away. I got his undivided attention. That was a first.

2. He took his time and asked me lots of questions — about me.

3. I had recent labs from all the other doctors, which he could interpret; they couldn't.

4. After looking at my history, he told me what I was feeling … and he was right on everything.

5. He knew what to do to give me my life back. Here I am not even five months later, and I'm feeling on top of the world.

   - No hot flashes.
   - I sleep better at night. I am sleeping.
   - I do not urinate ten times a night.
   - No nervous leg.
   - No joint pains.
   - I can wear wool.
   - I can wear makeup.
   - I do not cry, and I'm in charge of my emotions.
   - I can think again.
   - I can remember again.
   - Cholesterol is down and I'm off pills.
   - I AM STRONG
   - The list goes on and on.

"Dr. Lee, you are my hero. Please live your life carefully because, without you, I don't have a life.

"With much love, Paula Sommer" – Colorado, May 2011

* * *

"I am a mid-sixties psychologist and I plan to work in this field that I love until I am in my eighties. I took HRT in past years and noticed an emotional difference when I stopped. So about three years ago, I began using the cream offered by Dr. Lee's pharmacy. I have experienced a noticeable difference in my emotions, which I must keep stable in order to work effectively as a mental-health professional. An added benefit is that most people tell me I look five to ten years younger and they are surprised when they learn my age. I continue to exercise regularly, eat a healthy diet, and get adequate sleep; but the HRT has been a real bonus!!" – Dr. Patricia Covalt, Ph.D., LMFT, Colorado, May 2011, author *What Smart Couples Know*

The *Keys* to Women's Health

– Throughout Life!

Why Bioidentical Hormone Replacement Therapy?

The last time I checked, we do not have leaves. We are not plants. We are not horses, either. We need human estrogen, human progesterone, human testosterone, human DHEA, human thyroid, human insulin, etc. Plant-derived and horse-derived estrogens are not *natural* to the human body.

Every time, in medicine, we have tried animal hormones, we have had some type of trouble. Most studies on estrogen in humans have been done using *horse* estrogen (Premarin, or conjugated equine estrogen) and non-bioidentical, manufactured progesterone (Provera, or medroxyprogesterone acetate). Unfortunately, those studies have little to do with what wonders can be accomplished by using bioidentical hormones, which are synthesized from yams or soy, as a starting point. To say that all estrogens are alike is like saying all antibiotics are alike. There are profound differences in penicillins, tetracyclines, and sulfa drugs, for example.

The primary estrogen produced naturally in the ovaries is estradiol. The difference between estradiol and testosterone is miniscule — yet they perform quite differently in the body. Likewise, horse-derived estrogen and bioidentical estrogen have small differences, but they function profoundly differently in the body.

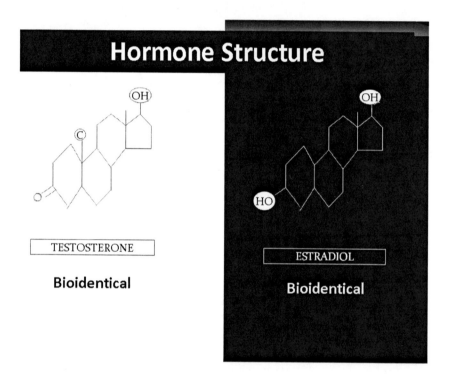

The differences in the chemical structure of testosterone and estrogen (estradiol) are subtle, yet significant. On the very left hand side of the molecule, notice that testosterone has a double bond to "O" (oxygen); whereas, estradiol has a single bond to an "OH" (oxygen and hydrogen, called a hydroxyl group). Also notice that testosterone has an extra "C" (carbon) atom above and between the first two rings. These are the only molecular differences between testosterone and estrogen.

"Biologically identical" hormones are available for estrogen, progesterone, testosterone, DHEA, growth hormone, thyroid, and so forth. The reason we don't see bioidentical hormones in the marketplace very much yet is that the pharmaceutical companies cannot patent a naturally occurring substance (meaning they cannot make big profits on these substances).

Bioidentical hormones naturally occur in menstruating women. They are synthesized in a lab setting from yam or soy. (If you think about it, it has to be synthesized; we cannot take young women's hormones.) What is important is that the resultant molecule is exactly the same as what the human body makes. They are twins. Your body recognizes a bioidentical hormone as "self", not a foreign invader. This synthesis is OK as long as it is done properly.

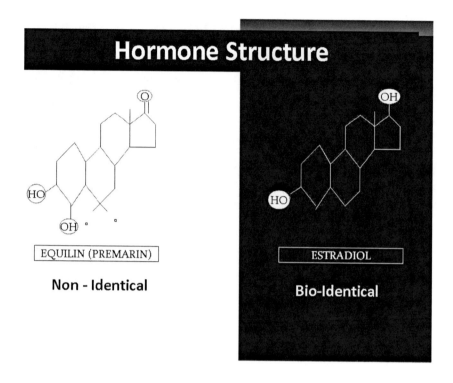

The differences in the molecular structure of Equilin, one of the major hormones in Premarin, and estradiol, the major human estrogen, are also small. Note that the "O" (oxygen) molecule at the very top of Equilin has a double bond; whereas, at the same position on estradiol, there is an "OH" (hydroxyl group) with a single bond. Also notice that Equilin has an "OH" at the bottom of the first ring; whereas, estradiol has nothing in that position. These differences in structure account for all the biological differences in function.

Menopause and Women's Hormones

Menopause is a normal event in women's lives, and it can be quite different for two different women. Technically, it is the total cessation of menstruation for one year, when the ovaries quit making estrogen, progesterone, and testosterone.

This hormone deficiency state often results in any of these annoying symptoms: night sweats, hot flashes, insomnia, fatigue, depression, moodiness, anxiety, vaginal dryness, vaginal odor, irritability, loss of sexual interest, hair growth on face, painful intercourse, panic attacks, weird dreams, urinary tract infections, vaginal itching, lower back pain, bloating, flatulence (gas), indigestion, osteoporosis, hair loss, frequent urination, snoring, sore breasts, palpitations, varicose veins, urinary leakage, dizzy spells, skin feeling crawly, migraine headaches, memory lapses; aching ankles, knees, wrists, shoulders, and heels — and just not feeling like yourself.

Not all women get all of these symptoms, and a few have none at all. Many of these symptoms may occur during "peri-menopause," the approximately one to five years leading up to the complete cessation of menstruation. The average age of menopause is fifty to fifty-one, but it can begin as early as thirty-five or as late as fifty-five.

When is it time to seek treatment for these symptoms? Or is treatment really necessary? Treatment is *very* necessary. What's been misconceived is the problems that result from *not* taking hormones. An insufficient level of hormones in the body allows diseases to sneak in and take over.

One recent study recommended antidepressants to cut down on hot flashes. That's ridiculous. Why take antidepressants, sleeping pills, cholesterol medications, all wrought with complications and side effects, when you can fix the entire problem by taking appropriate bioidentical hormones?

Estrogen

Estrogen has four hundred actions in a woman's body. The female body has receptor sites for estrogen on all of the cell membranes: in the brain, muscles, bone, bladder, gut, uterus, ovaries, vagina, breast, eyes, heart, lungs, and blood vessels.

How to Know If Your Body Has Enough Estrogen

If your estrogen level is low or deficient, you may experience some or several of these symptoms, but most likely not all: more wrinkles as the skin thins, vaginal dryness and itching, acne, oily skin; urinary tract infections and/or incontinence; reduced memory, cognition, mental clarity, physical dexterity, sexual interest, breast size; increased LDL cholesterol, and chance of diabetes; osteoporosis or osteopenia (a mild, less severe form of osteoporosis).

In addition to menopause, stress also suppresses estrogen function. It is actually cortisol excess depressing both estrogen and testosterone. Various methods of stress management may counter this.

Another factor that depletes estrogen is cigarette smoking. For women who smoke, the body's natural estrogen levels are lower (at any age). Smoking also increases the incidence of all cancers, including breast cancer; although the exact percentage has not yet been identified. If you smoke (and you are quitting), how much estrogen supplementation do you need? I would balance this according to the estrogen levels determined by your blood tests. If you are young and ovulating on your own, no supplementation would be given.

Some women have too much estrogen, although that is uncommon. Some of the more common symptoms of too much estrogen are heavy menstruation, bloating, vicious headaches, unusual fatigue and irritability, swollen and sensitive breasts, restless sleep, and decreased interest in sex. Additional symptoms to look for are depression with anxiety and agitation, panic attacks, unusual weight gain (especially around the middle). Less common symptoms, determined by medical diagnosis, may be hypothyroidism, uterine fibroids, fibrocytic breast disease. Excess estrogen, without counterbalancing progesterone, also can increase your risk of cancer of the uterus and breasts, as well as autoimmune diseases. So, getting the right balance of estrogen (and the right kind of estrogen) is critical for your health.

Although few women have too much estrogen, it can be due to a number of reasons, including: insufficient fiber and grains in the diet, overweight or obese, and/or no exercise. Too much estrogen also can occur with an overdose of supplemental estrogen. Impaired elimination of estrogen may occur if you are a poor methylator and your body does not detoxify estrogen properly; or you have chronic very poor health. Liver disease also may be a factor, which can be determined only by diagnostic tests. Another possible cause of excess estrogen is constipation, when excreted estrogen gets reabsorbed. Estrogen metabolites may be elevated with poor detoxification of estrogen, which is dependent upon hydroxylation and methylation. Environmental estrogens also may contribute to excess; such as high exposure to soy, pesticides, plastics and/or bisphenol A, which is in plastics and has become a huge problem. It is in plastic water bottles and it lines all cans.

The solution to all of these potential problems (too much estrogen; or, as in menopause, not enough) is proper testing. With the right balance of estrogen:

- You feel more energetic.

- Your memory and cognition return to normal.

- Your sleep is better and more renewing.

- You regain sexual interest and some libido.

- You are less easily irritated.

- Your weight issues improve. The proper amount (and kind) of estrogen supplementation increases your metabolism, which helps with weight maintenance and the ability to lose weight.

The right balance of estrogen also:
- Can help with fine motor skills, the production of nerve growth, and the prevention of tooth loss.

- It improves insulin sensitivity, which helps with blood sugar regulation.

- It keeps hot flashes and night sweats away, by regulating the body's temperature. (It is the absence or reduction of estrogen that brings on these symptoms.)

The benefits of the proper balance (and the right kind) of estrogen are crucial to your health — physically, mentally, and emotionally. Hormonal balance is critical!

Major Benefits of Estrogen Supplementation

1. *Supports Heart and Arteries*
New data by Jacque Rosseau, M.D. in the April 2007 issue of the *Journal of the American Medical Association* (*JAMA*) shows that women who take estrogen within ten years of

menopause reduce their risk of heart disease by 35 percent. This is huge, considering that heart disease is the leading cause of death for both women and men. This information was reaffirmed in a study by Andrea LaCroix, M.D., published in the April 2011 issue of the *Journal of the American Medical Association* (*JAMA*). Her 10.5 year follow-up on the women in the Women's Health Initiative (WHI) Premarin-only arm shows a nearly 50 percent reduction in heart disease, and a 23 percent reduction in breast cancer.

Estrogen also:

- Lowers blood pressure.

- Decreases lipoprotein; acts as a calcium channel blocker to keep arteries open.

- Dilates small arteries; helps to maintain their elasticity to help maintain blood pressure and to enhance cardiac function.

- Stimulates production of an enzyme that helps to prevent Alzheimer's.

- Decreases accumulation of plaque in arteries, and helps to stabilize plaque (to help prevent thrombosis).

- Inhibits platelet "stickiness," reducing the chance of heart attack or stroke and plaque formation in the arteries. (Platelets tend to adhere to what they are near: other cells, vessel walls, especially plaque and ruptured plaque, and to one another.) When plaque ruptures, for example, it is the platelets that adhere to it, probably trying to cover it over. However, this usually gets overdone and enough adherence occurs that the entire blood vessel becomes occluded.)

The KEEPS and KRONOS research studies, currently underway and expected to come out within the year, I believe will show that women taking estrogen, *as menopause begins,* prevents thickening of the lining of their blood vessels (intimal thickness), indicating that estrogen may help to prevent heart disease and stroke.

It is fair to emphasize that estrogen will not "save you" from a steady diet of fast food and potato chips. Although estrogen does reduce inflammation and risks associated with heart disease, it will not repair a damaged heart. Diet and exercise are still the essential pillars of health maintenance. In fact, one of the greatest factors in heart health is consistent and daily exercise, like walking.

2. *Sharpens Brain Function and Alertness*

Recent studies of brain function, at Stanford and Yale, employed computer programs to measure memory and cognition in postmenopausal women, divided into two groups: women taking estrogen, and those not taking estrogen. Those taking estrogen scored significantly higher in brain function. Estrogen:

- Gets rid of brain fog.

- Enhances reasoning, concentration, and problem-solving.

- Enhances memory.

- Is shown to enhance nerve cell growth.

3. *Corrects and Prevents Bone Loss (osteoporosis, osteopenia)*

Estrogen is the best substance for restoring bone density and preventing bone loss (osteoporosis). Without estrogen, as many as 30 to 50 percent of women are subject to a fracture — twenty to thirty years *after* menopause. This doesn't happen overnight, but it does happen. Only about half of women with a hip fracture live an additional year, so this is a very serious concern. Those who don't have a hip fracture may have painful compression fractures of the vertebra in the spine, which can be crippling. A woman's risk of a fracture in older age is greater than her risk of breast cancer!

Osteopenia is also the loss of bone, only less severe than osteoporosis. On a bone density scan, the report gives a T score. 0 to -1.0 is normal. Down to -2.5 is osteopenia. Below -2.5 is osteoporosis (e.g., -2.9 as in one patient). So, it is severity of disease in bone loss. One may have osteopenia first and progress to osteoporosis.

- Calcium alone does not prevent osteoporosis or osteopenia. (Most people don't get enough calcium in their diet, anyway.)

- A good second line of therapy for osteoporosis is SERMs (selective estrogen receptor modifier); such as, the drugs Fosamax, Boniva, Evista, Actonel. However, researchers are learning that SERMs may not be making the best kind of bone . . . and may be depleting bone in the jaw.

- The best treatments for bone strength and density, unequivocally, are estrogen, progesterone, and testosterone. All of these hormones occur naturally in the body; however, supplementation is needed during menopause and andropause, because the levels become too low. For additional very significant statistics and data on addressing osteoporosis and osteopenia, please see the comprehensive discussion in the Men's Manual in the section titled "Testosterone and Bones." It's there, because bone disease affects men, too.

- In addition, vitamins D_3 and K_2 are highly recommended for daily supplementation, because their levels are found to be almost routinely low when checked. Generally recommended: 2,000-6,000 units of D daily, 100 mcg for K_2, although these doses may vary to individual needs. These two vitamins bring the calcium from vegetables and dairy products into the bones; even though testosterone speeds up the rebuilding of bone, estrogen slows the reabsorption of bone. For the strongest bones and quickest results, the optimal quantity of D_3 depends upon the individual, so cutting-edge doctors monitor the level in the blood stream by testing. (Note: rarely you will find vitamin D_3 combined with vitamin K.)

- Exercise, especially weight-bearing, also strengthens the bones.

4. *Reduces the Risk of Colon Cancer*

Two studies, including the 2002 Women's Health Initiative, have shown that estrogen reduces the risk of colon cancer by as much as 40 percent (8 in 10,000). This is significant when we realize that colon cancer kills more women than breast cancer. Breast cancer is more frequent, but colon cancer is more lethal. Most women's greatest health risk is heart disease, but colon cancer is becoming a bigger killer than breast cancer. (Please also see the appendix "The Misleading 2002 Women's Health Initiative Report.")

5. *Smoothes Skin Elasticity*

In particular, estrogen diminishes wrinkles, which is why major cosmetics manufacturers add it to their products. I am not saying that estrogen prevents wrinkles, nor that it gets rid of wrinkles. It does promote thickening of the underlying connective tissue in the skin, which makes the skin look smoother, plumper, and softer. Estrogen enhances the collagen that supports and underlies the epidermis, giving the skin a healthier look.

Without hormones, the skin that lines the vagina atrophies and becomes thin and inelastic, and the women complain of dryness and itching. So, intercourse can become painful. Plus, these women are more susceptible to vaginal infections.

6. *Improves Bladder Function*

The bladder is very estrogen sensitive. Without estrogen, the bladder atrophies and loses elasticity, which makes it leakier and more prone to bladder infections.

7. *Prevents Vaginal Atrophy*

The vagina also is very estrogen sensitive. Without estrogen, it loses elasticity and becomes dry; this may cause abrasive discomfort during intercourse. Sometimes, vaginal walls crack and bleed. Without sufficient estrogen, the woman is also more prone to vaginal infections.

8. *Prevents Symptoms of Menopause*

Without sufficient estrogen, women may be plagued by any of these symptoms: hot flashes, night sweats, insomnia, mood swings, depression, and feeling as if bugs are crawling on you. These symptoms usually don't last forever, but they may be difficult for one to five years. Most doctors prescribe sleeping pills, antidepressants, and statin drugs — rather than *the real cure: hormones.* By the way, hot flashes are due to *fluctuating* levels of estrogen, not low levels.

9. *Mood*

Estrogen:

- Decreases depression, irritability, anxiety, pain sensitivity.

- Enhances energy.

- Improves mood.

- Improves sleep, which results in improved mood.

- Reverses the poor moods for which menopause is famous.

10. *Eyes*

Estrogen reduces the risk of cataracts, and protects against macular degeneration. It diminishes "dry eye," from which many menopausal women suffer.

Is Estrogen Supplementation Safe?

Yes, estrogen supplementation is safe — *and* necessary. *Bioidentical* estrogen supplementation is beneficial to continued health and well-being. It raises HDL cholesterol (healthy kind) by 10 to 15 percent, and lowers LDL cholesterol (unhealthy kind).

Estrogen has been put under incredible scrutiny in numerous studies. Other drugs, like high blood pressure meds, heart meds, even antibiotics, if put under similar scrutiny would not fare nearly as well. The issue of estrogen supplementation has lost perspective. When the average woman on the street is asked, "What is your greatest health risk?" today she usually replies "breast cancer." In fact, the answer is heart disease.

Nevertheless, there is much debate regarding estrogen and breast cancer. If one gets breast cancer, estrogen can speed its growth. However, in the 2002 Women's Health Initiative (WHI) study, one group of women were given only Premarin (horse estrogen); and that group of women had a *reduction* in breast cancer, not an increase. Furthermore, LaCroix's 10.5 year follow-up study on that group of women, published in the April 2011 issue of *JAMA,* reports that they have a 23 percent reduction in breast cancer.

*I do **not** believe estrogen causes breast cancer.* It is known, however, that a glass of wine daily quadruples one's risk of breast cancer, and being overweight doubles the risk. *Important note:* Exercise cuts *in half* the risk of breast cancer.

The only real risk of estrogen is that post-menopausal women who are taking the *oral* estrogen supplementation do have a four-fold increased risk of getting a blood clot. The 2007 French ESTER report, published in *Circulation,* clearly and convincingly showed that as long as estrogen is taken transdermally (through the skin, creams or patches), there is no increased risk of blood clots.

For example, the 2002 Women's Health Initiative study (WHI), performed by multiple centers (see appendix), reported that estrogen gives women breast cancer. This report frightened 70 percent of women in the United States and around the world into stopping their *protective* hormones . . . and it is still impacting medical decisions today, even though now all the findings of the WHI have been disproven by recent studies.

Even in the WHI report, the only estrogen used (Premarin, a horse estrogen) showed *no increase* in breast cancer. In fact, that report showed a *downward* trend, which some statisticians now say is a statistically significant decline in breast cancer among women taking only Premarin.

In 2003, after the WHI data had been analyzed, numerous OB-Gyn doctors, including Leon Speroff, M.D., a recognized authority on hormones and author of *Clinical Gynecologic Endocrinology and Infertility,* reported that some of the WHI findings were *not* statistically significant.

Most notable: There were two groups in the WHI study: one took a combination of horse-urine estrogen (Premarin) with an artificially manufactured progestin (Provera); another took only the horse estrogen and no progesterone. The group taking only the estrogen had *no* increased risk of breast cancer; whereas, the group taking the combination (Premarin and Provera) did have a small increased risk (8 in 10,000). *This leads me to question whether the artificially manufactured progesterone (progestin), in fact, might be the troublemaker causing breast cancer.*

In April 2007, the WHI *reversed their original finding.* The lead author, Jacque Rosseau, published in the *Journal of the American Medical Association* that they had "misinterpreted" some of the data (Rosseau, J.E., et al., *JAMA;* 297:1465–1477). They had looked at the data based on how many years after menopause the woman was during the study; particularly women within ten years of menopause, most in their fifties.

The new findings: Women who start estrogen within ten years of menopause have only a 1 or 2 out of 10,000 increased risk of breast cancer (the original WHI report had stated 8 out of 10,000, and that was using artificial Premarin and Provera).

Provera is now shown to be the problem with breast cancer (not estrogen). Provera is an artificial progesterone-like medication; it is *not* a healthy or a reliable substitute for bioidentical progesterone.

The 2007 *JAMA* article also reported that women who start estrogen within ten years of menopause *reduce* their risk of heart disease by 35 percent. This is tremendous news — because 53 percent of women die from heart disease, which is twelve times *more common* than death from breast cancer. This finding was even based on the horse-derived Premarin (pill). How much better would the data have been if the estrogen studied had been bioidentical, transdermal, and in an optimal dosing range determined by the individual patient's measuring blood levels?

In addition, these same women had *no* increased risk of stroke; the increased risk of breast cancer was minimized to 1-2 in 10,000; and the risk of colon cancer decreased by 6-8 in 10,000 (about a 36% reduction). Imagine the findings of a study on bioidentical hormones!

Not a single, large, double-blinded, cross-over, reputable study has shown conclusively that breast cancer is even related to estrogen, especially not to bioidentical estrogen. There remain too many questions. For example, if breast cancer is caused by estrogen, why do postmenopausal women who do not take estrogen still get breast cancer — in increasing numbers as they age? Why does the use of birth control pills (very high estrogen doses) *not* correlate with an increased risk of breast cancer? Why are there good studies that *do* show that women who do take estrogen *after* breast cancer have *less* recurrence than those who do not take it?

No studies have implicated estrogen as causing uterine cancer, either, when progesterone is also given to balance the estrogen. It *is* now standard medical practice for doctors to give progesterone along with estrogen, because it has been found that the combination statistically does lower the risk of uterine cancer. Likewise, the large and authoritative EPIC study out of Europe showed a *decreased* risk of breast cancer when progesterone was given with estrogen. In addition, LaCroix's 10.5 year follow-up study published in the April 2011 issue of *JAMA* confirms that women taking Premarin only (no Provera, the progestin) have a 23 percent reduction in breast cancer and a nearly 50 percent reduction in heart disease.

The fact is that more women die from colon cancer than from breast cancer. Breast cancer is more frequent, more common, but only 4 percent of women die from it. Colon cancer has a far worse outcome, frequently death.

The greatest killer of women actually is heart disease; 53 percent of women of all ages. So heart disease is a much greater concern — and estrogen is *proven* to reduce heart disease by 30-50 percent (that is 3,500 fewer cases of heart disease out every 10,000 women). This is very good news regarding hormonal replacement.

Important Points Concerning All Estrogen Studies To Date

Ninety-nine percent of *all* estrogen studies in the United States have been done using Premarin (horse-derived); which tells us nothing about estradiol, the bioidentical and human equivalent of estrogen. Also, the patients were never monitored to determine if they were receiving an appropriate dose to restore their normal levels of hormones. Plus, Premarin is comprised of several different estrogens, and the manufacturer has not even told us how many or what all is in Premarin. Just because Premarin was the most widely prescribed estrogen around the world in 2002 (controlling 70 percent of the market) doesn't mean the data from its usage should be extrapolated to apply to *all* forms of estrogen. Blaming all forms of estrogen for cancer is like thinking that because ampicillin may cause some diarrhea, all antibiotics should be outlawed. Both are ridiculous notions.

Estradiol (E2) is the most potent of estrogens. Estriol (E3) is eighty times *less* potent. You may hear claims that E3 prevents cancer. This is not proven. I think it is simply a matter of less potency. I recommend the bioidentical estrogen, estradiol, given transdermally (patch, cream) directly through the skin.

The only progesterones studied have been primarily progestins (Provera, medroxyprogesterone acetate; in a few cases, Norlutate, norethindrone acetate). These are progesterone-like *artificially manufactured chemical compounds.* Their behaviors in the body are in some important ways unlike that of bioidentical progesterone, which is synthesized from naturally occurring soy or yam, resulting in a molecule exactly like the human body makes.

Progestins have been shown to increase breast cancer risk; whereas bioidentical progesterone does not (see the French EPIC study). Progestins have a negative effect upon cholesterol, triglycerides, HDL, and LDl; bioidentical progesterone has a positive effect.

In addition, no study of which I know has measured the levels of hormones *in the blood stream.* This is a significant shortcoming of studies on hormones. A "one size fits all" therapy can cause an overdose or an underdose. Without knowing the individual patient's blood levels, and adjusting to optimal dosing, hormonal *studies* are not only inadequate, they are misleading. If estrogen and progesterone levels are not checked during a study, how can we know the percentage of patients overdosed or underdosed? We can't. We also cannot know whether an overdosed patient had all or most or none of the breast cancers reported. *Studying the wrong form of estrogen, and in the wrong dose, can lead only to the wrong conclusions.* Premarin (horse-derived) and bioidentical (estradiol) are not the same and have some different results in the body's functions.

The 2002 Women's Health Initiative (WHI) study did show a tiny shift (2 in 10,000) toward an increased risk of Alzheimer's. However, the study had many flaws. Over half the participants were obese (average body mass index 28.5); which correlates with an increased risk of dementia, cancer, heart disease, diabetes, and hypertension. Also, 50 percent of the study participants were past or present smokers, which presents an elevated risk of heart attack and many cancers. The average age of the participants, when they began taking hormones, was sixty-three. If there is any benefit to taking hormones, it was lost on these women because they started thirteen years too late. The lining of blood vessels thickens with age; whereas, with estrogen, there is little or no such thickening. The lack of estrogen until age sixty-three set up these participants for a greater risk of vascular disease, blood clots, plaque, and heart attack — which is exactly what the researchers found (and they seemed surprised).

Regarding the WHI report about the increased risk of blood clots from taking estrogen, this is not new. We've known this for forty to fifty years. However, *now* we are learning more about blood-clotting disorders, and we have lab capability to measure Factor V Leiden Deficiency, Anti-Thrombin III, Protein S, Protein C, Anti-Phospholipid Syndromes, etc., as well as a much greater ability to predict who might be at increased risk. One study found that if you exclude patients with Factor V Leiden Deficiency, there is almost *no* increased risk of blood clotting when taking estrogen.

Another interesting observation supported by studies is that there is a *less* increased risk of blood clots when using transdermal estrogen (patches, compounded creams, lozengers), compared to oral (pill) estrogen. Both a 2003 study reported in the prestigious journal *Lancet* (Scarabin, et al.; 362(9382): 428-32) and a 2007 ESTER French study reported in the publication *Circulation* (Canonico, et al.; 115: 840-845) found no increased risk using transdermal bioidentical estrogen, contrasted with oral estrogen that has a four-fold increased clotting risk.

Despite the WHI indicating that estrogen is not protective of the heart for women in their seventies, the study *did* show a 35 percent *decreased* risk of cardiovascular disease in women within ten years of menopause (Rosseau, J.E., et al., *JAMA*, 2007; 297:1465–1477). This is consistent with a preponderance of evidence in the literature that estrogen protects the heart; which is probably due to the long-term effects of estrogen lowering LDL (unhealthy cholesterol) and raising HDL (healthy cholesterol), as well as due to decreased intimal thickness, better dilatation of coronary blood vessels, and the positive effect on matrix metalo-proteinases. No one would expect estrogen to improve an already diseased heart, which was proven by the data in the older women who did not have the protection of estrogen after menopause. The 1998 HERS study, published in the *Journal of the American Medical Association* (*JAMA*), also showed that estrogen does not repair an already damaged heart.

Also, the WHI study's data on the occurrence of breast cancer was only 8 in 10,000 for women with an average age of sixty-three. For women within ten years of menopause (usually in their fifties), the risk was only 1 in 10,000. The time required for a cancer to grow large enough to be "discoverable" is *ten* years. Yet in the WHI study, breast cancers were identified at six and seven years into the study, meaning it was more likely that the women had microscopic undiscoverable breast cancers when they *entered* the study and the estrogen did *not* cause their breast cancers. (The cancers may have grown faster due to the estrogen, though.)

The 2003 and 2007 significant contradictions to the 2002 WHI study have not been reinforced in subsequent general medical literature, and certainly not in the lay press. So non-OB-Gyns who do not closely follow gynecology updates have not received the critical news that the 2002 WHI study was *flawed.* Many OB/Gyns are even unaware of the follow-up studies and published reports in 2003 and 2007. Doctors tend to study their own specialties. For example, my specialty is hormones. Unless a doctor specializes in an area regarding hormones, he or she most likely has not yet discovered that estrogen, in fact, now has been found to be beneficial to women's overall health. In other words, your family practitioner or internist may not know the latest information on hormonal treatments. In fact, there have been many conflicting studies. This is not to imply that these doctors do poor work. It is very difficult to keep up with all changes in medicine. I cannot keep up with all of the changes, for example, in pediatrics; so I refer pediatric questions to pediatricians.

I believe the 2002 WHI study and their proponents were very wrong. Many physicians today have come to believe that it is *estradiol,* not Premarin, that *reduces* the risk of breast cancer. That has not yet been proven in large, multi-center studies; however, lab work on the metabolic pathways of different estrogens leads me to believe this is true.

It is fair to say that estrogen has *some* risks. However, they are very small risks and are overstated. The use of Premarin and artificial progestin in the WHI study (rather than bioidentical hormones) made the results very misleading. Likewise, the "one size fits all" concept of hormone dosing also made the results of the study misleading.

Very few studies on bioidentical hormones and estradiol are currently being done, except for some excellent European studies like the EPIC and ESTER studies. Of those that have been initiated, the results will not be known for another few years. The current Kronos and KEEPS studies, nearly completed, are oriented more toward hormones and heart disease. The Europeans have been using bioidentical hormones decades longer than the United States, and also have been using transdermal delivery systems much longer. Thus, the Europeans have done many good studies on bioidentical hormones.

For more on the Misleading WHI Study, please see the appendix.

News Flash! 2010 October

I regret to tell you that the media has struck once again. The 2002 Women's Health Initiative study resurfaced again in the national news. Remember, the WHI study said that hormones are evil, bad, nasty — and almost everybody took this information hook, line, and sinker, including doctors and patients.

Leon Sperhoff, M.D., Professor Emeritus at Oregon Health Sciences Center; Phillip Sarrell, M.D., Professor Emertitus at Yale Medical School; and Wulf Utian, M.D., Professor Emeritus at Case Western Reserve Medical College and immediate past President of the North American Menopause Society, all have stated that the information from the WHI report is *misleading* and basically *inaccurate.*

You can see the true facts with your own eyes in a new documentary, *Hot Flash Havoc.* This 2011 feature film documents that the WHI study was flawed. As I stated earlier, it was a study of women with (1) an average age of sixty-three (ten years too late for an accurate study), who were (2) obese and also (3) smokers. Furthermore, all the patients were given the *pill* forms; plus, it was Premarin (horse estrogen) and Provera (artificially manufactured look-alike progesterone). Participants were not given any bioidentical hormones.

As written earlier, Provera now has been strongly linked to increased risk of breast cancer. Whereas, bioidentical progesterone is linked to a *lack* of risk of breast cancer. So, the WHI link to increased risk of hormones is basically false! Even so, the media has reported all this as true.

I cannot say there is no risk, which I discuss below — but it is safe to say that the risk is minimal.

We must stick with bioidentical hormones (estrogen, progesterone, testosterone, DHEA, thyroid; estrogen transdermal, or through the skin). Again, I use transdermal unless for various reasons it doesn't work for some individual. Plus, I always work toward finding the optimal dose for each person, checking and rechecking the lab values if necessary, because each person is different. I use individualized dosing to obtain the optimal dosing for everyone.

I am absolutely convinced that bioidentical hormones *reduce* the risk of heart disease by at least 35 percent, colon cancer also by about a third, breast cancer by 23 percent, and bone loss by 40 percent.

We are reducing your risk of osteoporosis to almost zero. Without hormones, 40 percent of women are at risk of a fracture about thirty years after menopause. Only 40 percent of "little old ladies" with a fracture survive another year. This is very significant.

On bioidentical hormones, the brain works better, too. You have improved memory and cognition. The skin is fuller and smoother (fewer wrinkles). Women routinely sleep better and have more energy, better moods and quality of life. Hormones alleviate many health problems.

Having started as a medical doctor, then transitioned into the more specific study and research of bioidentical hormonal therapies, I am absolutely confident that they are not only safe but are critical for women's continued mental, emotional, and physical health and vitality.

Risks of Estrogen Supplementation

You Are In or Are Post Menopause

Nothing in this world is totally safe. Water is essential to life, yet too much at once in the wrong way can kill you. Oxygen is essential to life, yet too much at the wrong time (like for a newborn) can blind you. Sugar is essential to life, yet too much for too long results in diabetes and inflammation, which eventually will kill you.

I cannot say that taking estrogen, in any form, is riskless. But it is a *relatively* small risk, and there are so many benefits! Greater than the risk of taking estrogen is the risk to your general health if you do not replace hormones as they fade in the body with age.

Another major risk of estrogen replacement, even taken with progesterone, is the risk of *blood clot.* The 2007 ESTER study in France showed that postmenopausal women on a pill form of estrogen have a four-fold increased risk of blood clot and thromboembolic disease (blood clot that embolizes, such as to the lung). This is the same as the data on blood clotting collected during the Women's Health Initiative (WHI) study (and they were all pill takers). When using transdermal patches and creams, *no increased risk* of blood clots was reported, however. In fact, the ESTER study found that women taking estrogen transdermally through the skin (patch, cream, lozenge/troche made by a compounding pharmacist) actually have a *zero* (0) increased risk of a blood clot (Canonico, et al., *Circulation,* 2007; 115: 840-845). If one factors out the 5 percent of women with Factor V Leiden Deficiency (genetic increased risk of blood clots), there is very little if any increased risk of blood clot. In addition, the study reported, women on a pill form of estrogen have increased C Reactive Protein, which is associated with increased risk of heart attack and Alzheimer's.

When thinking of blood clots and increased risk, realize also that a blood clot in the heart is called a "heart attack," and a blood clot in the brain is called a "stroke." So clotting risk is a very significant risk.

Certainly, with these more recent 2003 and 2007 studies, it seems quite apparent that the data now show safety with bioidentical hormones, which are taken directly through the skin into the blood stream.

You Have Had Breast Cancer

You previously have had or overcome breast cancer and have been advised to avoid all estrogen and progesterone supplementation. Can you, or should you, take bioidentical estrogen and/or progesterone supplementation?

This is highly, highly controversial. Most doctors and breast cancer doctors will tell you, "Do not take estrogen." We fear that estrogen might make any remaining cancer cells grow.

However, recently, more and more breast cancer specialists are allowing patients to apply some estrogen vaginally; and some are allowing women to take estrogen when they are five years cancer free. Nevertheless, this does have to be an individual, case-by-case, decision.

People like Suzanne Somers, after careful consideration, and after carefully seeking out cutting-edge doctors, take regular doses of estrogen after having had breast cancer. Suzanne is a great example of a woman doing very well with her cancer. There actually are two or three studies showing that women on estrogen after breast cancer actually have *less* recurrence than women who avoid estrogen. These studies are in the minority, but they do exist.

What seems very promising is data showing that estrogen does *not* cause cancer. What may be confusing is that, although it may not *cause* cancer, if you already have breast cancer, taking estrogen could accelerate the growth. So doctors are cautious not to prescribe estrogen supplementation without regular diagnostic tests.

Thermograms have become a popular diagnostic tool. However, the best radiological minds are very concerned about these; because the findings cannot be replicated day after day, exam after exam, and the results do not correlate well to other diagnostic modalities.

Annual mammograms are still considered highly significant for early diagnosis. The U.S. has vastly superior statistics for breast-cancer survival, compared to other countries, as a result of yearly mammograms (starting at age 40). In women early diagnosed through mammograms, approximately 95 percent survive breast cancer. In addition, despite what you might have heard from media reports on some misguided governmental studies, mammograms are *not* dangerous; the radiation exposure is minimal. So, do not be fooled. Annual mammograms can save your life.

In addition to diagnostic tests if you already have breast cancer or a strong family history of it, nutriceuticals are shown to help deactivate estrogen in the body's tissues. For example, during the body's natural detoxification process, excess estrogen gets changed from a potent promoter of cell proliferation (including cancer cells) into a quiescent metabolite that does not cause cell proliferation. This change occurs in two steps: *step 1* hydroxylation (encouraged by the use of di-indole methane, or DIM, which can be found in health food stores); and *step 2* methylation (enhanced by taking a "methylator" such as methyl-B$_{12}$, methyl folate, trimethyl glycine, or SAMe). Another option is NAC (n-acetyl-cysteine), which deactivates estrogen during step 2 and is also a great antioxidant. Taking DIM or Indole-3-Carbynol to accelerate the hydroxylation, and a "methylator" to accelerate the methylation, also will aid in preventing breast cancer.

Perhaps even more vital to know, there is a building body of statistical research that *bioidentical* progesterone may *inhibit* breast-cancer cell growth. So, as explained throughout this book, my first recommendation for preventing breast cancer is always bioidentical hormones.

Progesterone

The menstrual years are a dance of estrogen and progesterone ebbing and flowing. The first half of the menstrual cycle is predominated by estrogen, with levels getting up to around 150-200 pg/ml. Progesterone during this phase is very low, at 1-4 ng/ml. Ovulation occurs at approximately mid-cycle, when estrogen peaks at around 400-500 pg/ml. Then progesterone becomes dominant, reaching levels of 15-25 ng/ml. Meanwhile, estrogen declines to around 200-250 pg/ml. Toward the end of the cycle, both hormones drop and, without hormonal support for the lining of the uterus, menstruation ensues. Progesterone is an essential balancing ingredient in this process.

It is important to balance the use of both estrogen and progesterone, because progesterone undoes any potential negative side-effects of estrogen taken alone. It now has been determined that progesterone does stop estrogen from causing uterine cancer. Also, more and more evidence indicates that it inhibits the initiation of breast cancer.[4] See the appendix "Progesterone and Breast Cancer Risk" for more information on progesterone studies.

Progesterone is also essential to a healthy female body. In addition to its important role in the menstrual cycle and in pregnancy, more and more studies are showing that this important GABA-like hormone:

- Calms the brain.

- Decreases depression.

- Helps with more restful sleep.

- Reduces foggy brain (clearer thinking).

- Fights weight gain.

- Fights diabetes.

---

[4] Fournier et al., Breast Cancer Research Treatment 2008;107:103; Fournier A, et al. *Breast Cancer Res Treat.* doi10.1007/S10549-007-9523-x.

- Decreases osteoporosis.

- Decreases immune system disorders.

- Helps to reduce hair loss.

- Enhances libido.

- Even reduces seizures and tremors.

Low Natural Progesterone in the Body

Menopause is the foremost cause of low progesterone. Other causes may be: sugar, excess saturated fat, excessive stress or cortisol, antidepressant medications, thyroid deficiency, excess arginine, increased lactation (prolactin hormone), low luteinizing hormone; deficiency in vitamins A, B$_6$, C, and/or zinc.

Symptoms that may indicate low natural progesterone in the body: excessive menstruation, inflammation, pain, osteoporosis, decreased HDL cholesterol; increased irritability, nervousness, moodiness, poor sleep, depression or prolonged deep sadness or lethargy, excessive weepiness or emotional distress. When you have multiple symptoms, the best way to know if you are low in progesterone is through a blood test by a lab.

In menopausal women, to mimic the physiology of earlier years, progesterone can be given for only the last two weeks of the cycle; however, menstruation would continue. Most women feel that one of the benefits of menopause is that the periods are finally over. So another way to handle progesterone is to take a lower dose daily, to achieve blood levels of 3-6 ng/ml. The low dose is necessary to avoid raising the cortisol; which tears down muscle, ligament and bone, and puts on fat, especially around the middle.

Artificially Manufactured Progesterone or Bioidentical?

Both bioidentical progesterone and progestins build bone density, help thyroid function, normalize copper and zinc levels in the body, protect against uterine cancer and fibrocystic breast disease.

Progestin is the artificially manufactured molecule that has some progesterone-like activity — but is *not* identical to progesterone. In the 2002 Women's Health Initiative (WHI) study, in which the two groups of women received the same estrogen (Premarin), one group received estrogen only; the other group received the artificially manufactured progestin (Provera) with their estrogen. The group that received the estrogen only had *no* increased risk of breast cancer; the group that also received the artificial progestin did have increased breast cancer.

For bioidentical progesterone (biologically identical to what is produced in the human body), pharmaceutical manufacturers also synthesize these hormones. They accomplish this by starting the process with a yam or soy product, then modify the molecule into a final product that is compatible to the human body and results in an exact match to what the body produces.

See the photos below. The first compares the molecular configuration of progesterone vs. the molecular configuration of Provera.

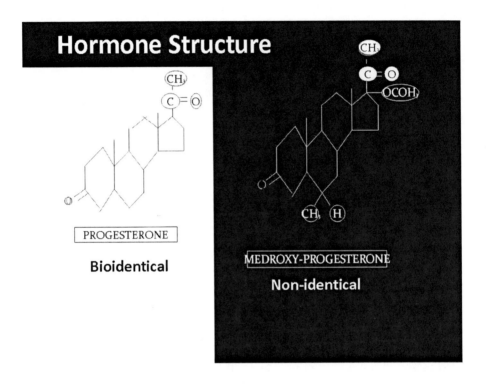

Notice that, compared to the bioidentical progesterone on the left, medroxyprogesterone (MPA) has additional "OCOH" at the top of the fourth ring, plus an extra "C" on the lower part of the second ring, accounting for the differences in how these molecules function.

So it seems that artificial progesterone (progestin) may be the cancer-producing factor, rather than estrogen in any form, as previously has been believed by the medical world.

By contrast, studies show that bioidentical progesterone, which is synthesized from yam or soy, does *not* increase the risk of breast cancer. In fact, it appears to be protective of breasts. We are waiting for confirmatory studies. For recent study results, please see the appendix "Progesterone and Breast Cancer Risk."

Side Effects of Progesterone Supplementation

The side effects from progestins (artificial) do *not* occur with bioidentical progesterone. Progestin side effects may include an increase in: weight, appetite, bloating, headache, poor sleep, irritability, restlessness, nervousness, depression, increased LDL cholesterol, increased risk of breast cancer. Other side effects of progestin may be: spotting, rash, acne, nausea, hair loss, tender breasts, loss of interest in sex, decreased energy, and decreased HDL cholesterol.

In addition, progestins do not help to balance estrogen. It can cause spasm in coronary arteries. It stops the protective effects of estrogen on the heart. It counteracts many of the positive effects of estrogen.

On the cautionary side, a few women are less tolerant of progestin supplementation and don't like the way they feel when they get too much. This is usually from the artificially manufactured pill form, of which the liver can metabolize only 80 percent of the dose, creating a negative effect upon the blood sugar and insulin and an adverse effect upon diabetic women. (Even non-diabetic women have an increased risk of developing diabetes later in life.)

With progestin, it is also difficult to determine the precise dose for each person. Too much progestin increases: appetite and craving of carbs, cortisol and fat storage, and insulin resistance. It suppresses the immune system and decreases insulin, glucose tolerance, and growth hormone. Symptoms you especially don't want are: urinary incontinence; feeling bloated, full, constipated; relaxed ligaments and/or muscles of the gut (because relaxed ligaments lead to joint injury and pain); low-back pain, achy legs and hips. If you are having multiple, chronic or extreme symptoms like these, the only way to know for sure how much supplemented progestin you are absorbing and need is with a blood test and to measure for an optimal level. However, progestin cannot be measured routinely. This is another disadvantage of trying to use progestin when progesterone is the better, and healthier, choice.

Benefits of Biologically Identical Progesterone

The benefits of biologically identical progesterone are numerous! It is the safest form of progesterone and has the greatest benefits:

- Balances the menstrual cycle and estrogen levels.

- Increases metabolism.

- Helps your body eliminate fats.

- Lowers cholesterol.

- Lowers blood pressure.

- Improves sleep.

- Improves memory.

- Increases the beneficial effects of estrogen.

- Increases scalp hair.

- Normalizes libido.

- Is a natural diuretic and antidepressant.

- Calms anxiety.

- Decreases the rate of cancer in receptors all over the body.

  Note: Your progesterone levels can be easily obtained in routine lab work.

You Have Had Your Uterus Removed

The risk of breast cancer is inhibited by progesterone. Bioidentical progesterone is still needed if one has no uterus, to protect against an increased risk of breast cancer with estrogen alone.

Testosterone

If estrogen and progesterone are the "cake," testosterone is the "icing." Most women really like the way they feel with a small addition of some testosterone. They report an increase in energy, vigor, vitality, and mental clarity.

Many studies on testosterone show an increase in bone mass, strengthening of the heart, vaso-dilation of coronary blood vessels, and decrease in blood sugar levels. Testosterone helps to clear thinking (rather than live with foggy brain). It aids in building strong bones, may aid in the maintenance of muscle, is somewhat protective of the breasts, and diminishes breast pain. It also enhances libido, which most menopausal women complain they have lost.

One woman began using testosterone cream at age sixty-three. She has noticed increased mental acuity, creative brainstorming and creative drive, a restored interest in creative activities and the ability to follow-through on projects. She says that testosterone supplementation "saved" her mind, when estrogen and progesterone were no longer enough. Despite years on hormone replacement therapy (pill forms of estradiol and medroxyprogesterone), she had lost mental concentration and ability to work (writer) as efficiently as in the past. Month to month, she noticed significant increases in mental capacity. At six months, she wrote an original screenplay, with the same clarity and vigor as pre-menopause.

Benefits of Testosterone Supplementation

Typical reported benefits of testosterone supplementation in post-menopausal women:

- Increased energy

- Muscle strength

- Sense of well-being

- Clearer memory

- Reduced breast sensitivity

- Body more toned (so skin sags less)

- Decrease in excess fat

- Decrease in bone loss (possibly even strengthening and restoring bone density)

- May increase libido (in 80 to 90 percent of women).

Symptoms of Possible Testosterone Deficiency

Particular symptoms of testosterone deficiency may be:

- Loss of pubic hair

- Loss of muscle tone

- Muscle wasting

- Droopy eyelids

- Sagging cheeks

- Thin lips

- Dry and thin skin

- Thinning hair.

More common symptoms include:

- Decreased sex drive

- Less dreaming

- Hyper-emotional states

- Hyper-anxious

- Fatigue

- Mild depression

- Low self-esteem

- Decreased HDL cholesterol

- Weight gain.

When you notice many of these symptoms occurring, or you are having particularly strong experiences, the best way to know if testosterone loss is a factor is to have a blood test.

Sometimes, low testosterone is perceived as a lack of energy. Typical causes of low testosterone levels include: childbirth, menopause, surgical menopause (ovaries removed), depression, trauma, and stress in general. Causes also may be: birth-control pills, cholesterol-lowering medications (statins), endometriosis, chemotherapy, and adrenal exhaustion.

Most women are deficient in testosterone, even before they are menopausal. Women's decline in this hormone starts at around age thirty-five to forty. Often testosterone is the first hormone to decline in women. Sometimes, it is helpful to lighten the burden of the hormonal transition by giving testosterone *before* a woman is deeply into menopause.

Being one of the hormones that declines with menopause, we need to restore the levels of *all* hormones to optimal levels, so they can do their work to maintain balance and heal the body and mind. All hormones work together synergistically, meaning that 1 + 1 + 1 is *greater than* 3.

How Lifestyle May Balance Your Testosterone Level

In addition to replacing diminished testosterone, changes in lifestyle help.

- In particular, increase protein and decrease simple carbohydrates (candy, chocolate, pie, cake, ice cream, fruit juices).

- Another key factor is daily exercise (walk 20-30 minutes a day).

- To reduce your stress (and lower cortisol), get enough sleep every night (adults over the age of twenty-six, 7-9 hours).

- To lose weight (lower cortisol), reduce your calorie intake by 20 to 30 percent daily.

- To naturally increase your body's production of testosterone on its own, take 10 to 20 mg of zinc, if you are deficient (most women and men are). Plus, take these amino acids:

  - *Arginine* − Abundant in chocolate, coconut, dairy, meats, oats, peanuts, soybeans, walnuts, wheat, wheat germ. Regulates the body's production of growth hormone. Releases insulin. Produces vasopressin (has to do with blood pressure). Strengthens immune system. Or supplement about 5 grams daily.

  - *Leucine* – In brown rice, beans, nuts, whole wheat. Helps to regulate blood sugar, the growth and repair of muscle. Enhances growth hormone production. Aids in wound healing.

- *Glutamine* – In beef, beans, poultry, fish, eggs, dairy. Important in building and maintaining muscle, enhancing the immune system. The source of fuel to the cells lining the intestine. Necessary for normal brain function. Or supplement 54 grams.

How to Take Testosterone Supplementation

Take as a transdermal cream, lozenge or troche, or as a pellet under the skin (patch not yet available, but a company is seeking FDA approval). Do not take orally (pill). Testosterone cannot be given as a pill because it can be toxic to the liver.

Typically, and most often, testosterone is prescribed as a cream, sometime a troche (better known as a lozenge). The disadvantage of troches is that they rapidly absorb by the cheeks, gums, and tongue, so the level races up too high; the hormone is then rapidly metabolized and degraded, so the level drops in two to three hours until the next dose in twelve to twenty-four hours.

Creams last in the blood stream many more hours, perhaps fourteen to sixteen hours. This gives a much more even release and a steady feeling in the patient. The dose is low enough that it is a very small amount of cream; such as 0.1 ml. that can easily be applied to the hairless area of the wrist, or behind the knee. Some people recommend that it be applied occasionally to the labia or clitoris, to enhance sexual response (this cannot be applied regularly or it might result in clitoral enlargement).

One could use intramuscular injections, but with the possibility to achieve adequate levels with something as simple as a cream, injections are not very inviting to most.

Symptoms of Excess Testosterone

Symptoms of excess testosterone in a woman (very rare) may include: hair loss, unwanted hair growth, infertility, irregular periods, anger, agitation.

Additional more common symptoms may be: salt and sugar cravings, hypoglycemia, acne, oily skin, weight gain, fluid retention, changes in memory, mood swings, depression, anxiety, fatigue, decreased HDL cholesterol, and increased insulin resistance. These more common symptoms are rare: Women worry that testosterone is going to make them grow hair, or lower their voice, or give them big muscles. None of these things happen.

If you experience many of these symptoms, or have strong experiences, always get a blood test to verify your hormonal levels and help to determine the source(s) of the symptoms.

To lower excess testosterone, take saw palmetto (300 mg) or zinc. This is extremely rare in women, as almost all menopausal women are very low in testosterone. However, you can avoid these symptoms with appropriate and measured doses of bioidentical testosterone.

Risks of Testosterone Supplementation

There are really no risks with testosterone as long as you don't take too much. Women are prescribed 1/100th of what a man is prescribed. Estrogen in adequate doses is needed with testosterone, because testosterone given alone may increase the risk of heart disease and breast cancer.

In the very small doses used, there is little risk. Women receive only 1-2 mg (men 200-300 mg). This very small dose for women is not enough to lower the voice or stimulate hair growth. Some women are more sensitive than others and might develop oily skin or acne. If that occurs, simply reduce the dose.

When we measure testosterone, we look at both the "total testosterone" and the "free testosterone." It is this free fraction of the total testosterone that is active and used by the body. So, we monitor both levels to evaluate what you need. Thus, as with estrogen and progesterone, the idea is to replenish what is missing in the body due to menopause — and bring your body back into balance.

Women like how they feel on testosterone supplementation. They tell me about how they have more energy, clearer thinking, and the return of a normal libido, which is the "icing on the cake" for most. Testosterone is very safe for use by women, and it is easy to use.

In closing this Women's Guide, my strong belief and recommendation is that bioidentical hormone supplementation is key to your best and lasting health, today.

The benefits of bioidentical hormones are simply remarkable:

- Decreases risk of the number one killer of both women and men, heart disease;

- Preserves and guards bones against osteoporotic fractures;

- Restores the brain, memory, and cognitive functions;

- Smoothes wrinkles and plumps the skin; and

- Stops those pesky menopausal symptoms like hot flashes and night sweats, loss of libido, insomnia, headaches, fuzzy brain, loss of memory, weight gain, aches and pains!

When a new patient comes in with a list of medications prescribed by a hurried, uninformed family doctor, I believe she needs none of these. Rather than a sleeping pill, antidepressant, cholesterol-lowering drug, bone-sparing drug, maybe something for high blood pressure; she needs her hormones balanced, a few supplements, better nutrition, and some form of light, easy exercise.

I guarantee you, these healthier and more natural treatments *will* result not only in vastly improved health but also clearer thinking, increased libido, restored energy, and an overall feeling of balanced well-being.

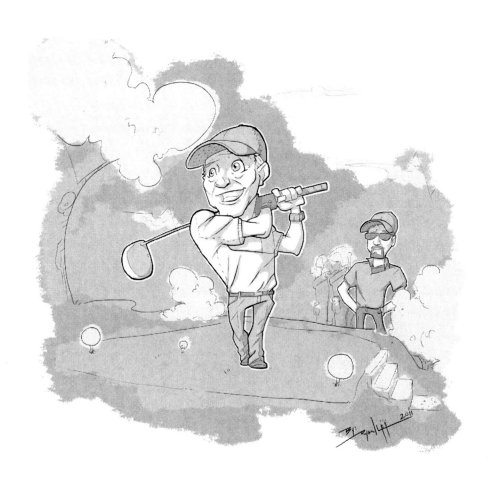

Illustration by Ryan Lee

The Men's Manual

Recapturing Your Vitality!

"I am a fifty-four-year-old male who started seeing Dr. Lee in April 2010. My wife informed me of his male Age Management practice, and what I read on his website seemed very interesting, so I made an appointment.

"Based on my first blood-test results, I didn't even begin to realize how much I needed his help and advice. I was overweight, diagnosed with Type 2 Diabetes, had high cholesterol, and was headed for a heart attack that could have very negative consequences. Dr. Lee was very caring and concerned, but he informed me that if lifestyle changes weren't made, and made quickly, I most likely would have those very negative consequences.

"He immediately put me on a vitamin regimen, gave me medicine to work on my diabetes, informed me of the glycemic index for controlling sugar in the foods I eat, and suggested that I exercise each day.

"As of six months later, I had lost thirty pounds, reduced my cholesterol from over 190 to 140 (HDL, the good stuff is climbing), lowered my blood sugar and, generally, was on the road to much better health. I follow his 'life changing' recommendations, even though I have much more to do. I am thankful that I have a doctor like him to guide and mentor me and be such a terrific supporter. I highly recommend Dr. Lee's Age Management practice to any man facing the challenges I did.

"Thanks, Dr. Lee. I look forward to continued progress under your care!" – Kent Rogers, Denver, Colorado, Sept. 2010

* * *

"When I first went to Dr. Lee, I was fifty-five and in good shape, but something was missing. The fire was gone, and it was reflected in my body. I worked out endlessly, but could never gain any muscle mass and I was turning into a pear. My wife suggested that I go to Dr. Lee and, even though he is an OB-GYN, he had expanded his practice to both menopausal women and andropausal men — because *he* was experiencing the same issues. Dr. Lee has made it his mission not only to help the ladies; he wants to help us guys, too, from the effects of aging.

"I went through the anti-aging program and, within several months, I was in a much better mood, my workouts were not only good but I could see the results. I felt better about life and I started chasing my wife of thirty years around again. Dr. Lee explained to me that this program would not prolong my life, but it will certainly make my life more enjoyable. And he was absolutely correct." – Richard Champion, age 59-½, Littleton, Colorado, May 2011

Men's Mid-Life Hormonal Needs

Testosterone

Men have been overlooked completely in the hormone arena. We know, without a doubt, that men's testosterone levels decline with age, and that men develop symptoms analogous to women's menopausal symptoms.

Testosterone replenishment is just as important to men's bodies as estrogen is to women's bodies. Men who lack sufficient testosterone levels are more prone to heart disease, prostate cancer, diabetes, mental confusion, Alzheimer's disease, bone loss (osteoporosis), muscle loss and frailty. Some men get very symptomatic, including hot flashes. They don't talk about it, because they think they're unusual. They aren't.

With the increasing depletion of testosterone, men lose energy, vitality, focus, sexuality, competitive spirit, and the will to win. Fat starts sticking, especially around the middle. Muscle tone drops, and workouts no longer get the same results. Some men get "brain fog," like women do in menopause. All of these are easily treated.

Replacing testosterone makes a phenomenal difference for 90 percent of men — and it is so easy to do. Testosterone replacement in men increases lean body mass, energy, sexual prowess, and the general feeling of well-being. Also, cortisol decreases — think *decreased stress.*

The typical male patient I see has the following type of story. In mid-life, men experience the onset of a lack of desire for work, sex, play, even hobbies. We begin losing muscle mass and strength. We lose interest in sex and don't perform as well, so sex becomes less satisfactory; some men think they need a new partner or an exciting escapade and their marriage may falter. Some men become grouchy, irritable or angry; some become depressed. For some, it's difficult to get a good night's sleep. Some experience joint or back pain, at least increased general aches and pains. Some men even get hot flashes.

We begin gaining a few pounds. Over a few years, the weight gain becomes twenty, thirty, forty pounds, and our clothes don't fit right. We may continue to work out, but the results are less effective. So, we become complacent and less competitive. We lose endurance and stamina. We lose our edge. With all of this going on, our self-image takes a nose dive and we become a couch potato.

No man escapes reduced testosterone production. Exercise helps to maintain some level of testosterone, but it eventually falls. This loss of testosterone level in men is called **andropause,** the male version of the female menopause (loss of estrogen). Men begin losing testosterone (1%-2% per year) beginning around age thirty-five to forty. By the time we are fifty or fifty-five, our testosterone level is about half what it was in our twenties.

Is the concept of andropause (male "menopause") a new unheard-of concept? No. Andropause was first studied and written about in 1944. In that study, "The Male Climacteric, Its Symptomology, Diagnosis, and Treatment," published in the *Journal of the American Medical Association*, Carl G. Heller showed the reversibility of andropause symptoms with treatment of testosterone supplementation. There have been hundreds of studies since that time.

Women lose their estrogen levels in only one to three years, making it a noticeable change. However, men lose their testosterone level gradually, 14 to 20 percent *per decade* (that's only 1%-2% *per* year). It's going on all the time; the change is so slow, that most men don't see it or feel it. Nonetheless, it *is* definitely happening. It is as difficult to notice as seeing your own children grow and change, even though they are changing daily.

Think back to your drive, stamina, endurance, vitality, concentration, and sexuality when you were twenty or twenty-five. Do you see a difference in you between now and then? Many men say it's only aging. That is correct! That is the point! You *can* maintain your health, vitality, vigor, stamina, memory, and sexual function your *entire* life when you employ the principles of Age Management, as spelled out in this Men's Manual.

Andropause is the most significant and anti-climatic time in a man's life. It comes on stealthily, slowly, and surely. I have now measured testosterone levels in hundreds of men. Without exception, those still in good health, with good vitality and normal brain function, good memory and cognition, have normal testosterone levels. The healthiest of them have testosterone levels in the high normal ranges. The higher the level, the better the men function.

If a man in your life (brother, husband, father, son) has unusual behaviors or symptoms, please inform him that he can achieve great advantage through hormone therapy; in combination with nutrition, supplements, glycemic index, stress management, adequate sleep, exercise in moderation; and reducing alcohol, nicotine, caffeine, and refined sugars.

Every cell in the body responds to and is regulated by hormones. So, as testosterone diminishes, our cells and organs go into chaos and our body doesn't function well. Our digestion is off. Our immune system works poorly, so we get more colds or flu. Our lungs don't give us oxygen as efficiently. Our heart and circulation systems are stressed by the increased weight and more plaque; whereas, testosterone supplementation can help to rebuild the heart muscle and dilate the coronary blood vessels.

Hormones, or their shortage, affect everything about how the body and brain work. Optimal functioning of every cell depends upon optimal hormonal levels. When the hormonal levels are no longer optimal, the body's organs and cells no longer function optimally. We have diminished abilities and diminished energy. Our entire health and well-being suffer.

Symptoms of low testosterone in men include: erectile dysfunction, decreased libido, increased fat mass (especially belly fat), increased insulin resistance (e.g., Type 2 Diabetes), decreased bone density (osteoporosis, even in men), long-term depression, and/or chronic fatigue.

Even the brain is adversely affected by testosterone loss. We have difficulty pulling up the names of people we know, difficulty retrieving facts, difficulty learning new things. Our quality of life is shrinking! We have entered the fuzzy, awkward, unpleasant stage of life!

Benefits of Testosterone Replacement in Men

Young men have a tremendously competitive spirit, a desire to be first and to outperform the competition. As we age, that competitive spirit wanes and we miss it, because competition has its place in the business environment and in leadership.

Replenishing the testosterone level in men is as important as replenishing estrogen and progesterone in women. Men notice a return of energy, vitality, and vigor, which are quite welcomed! Testosterone replacement therapy:

- Improves erectile dysfunction and libido.

- Increases drive, ambition, and energy.

- Increases lean body mass and weight loss.

- Improves muscles, strength, and bones.

- Improves memory and cognition.

- Reduces foggy brain and depression.

- Lowers blood sugar and the stress hormone cortisol.

- Reduces the risks of prostate cancer and heart attack.

- Strengthens the heart.

Testosterone and Heart Disease

Heart disease is caused by more than cholesterol. Blood sugar and diabetes also play a huge role. Even more overlooked is testosterone.

Cardiovascular disease (heart disease) is the number one killer of both men and women. Testosterone works to protect men's hearts, similarly to how estrogen protects women's hearts. Yet testosterone is a very overlooked area in men's health. Usually, when heart disease is mentioned, the next thought for men is cholesterol — yet half of heart attack victims have a normal cholesterol level.

Testosterone does help the heart in many ways. It builds and strengthens the muscle of the heart. It is the body's strongest factor in maintaining protein, particularly in the muscles. More than any other organ in the body, the heart is filled with testosterone receptors, indicating the importance of this hormone for the heart.

Testosterone stimulates the production of nitric oxide, an extremely potent dilator of blood vessels, including the coronary vessels; testosterone increases the power of the pump, which makes the heart more efficient. Medical journals report a high correlation between high testosterone and *low* heart disease in men.

Testosterone provides these benefits to the cardiovascular system:

- Lowers blood pressure.

- Lowers cholesterol and triglyceride levels, decreasing the risk of arterial plaque.

- Decreases insulin, by helping to lower blood sugar.

- Decreases lipoprotein.

- Decreases estrogen levels, lowering stroke and heart attack risks.

- Decreases visceral fat, belly fat, which decreases the risk of heart problems.

- Decreases the stress hormone, cortisol.

- Decreases fibrinogen; therefore, the risk of blood clots.

- Increases nitric oxide, which dilates blood vessels and increases heart blood flow.

- Increases energy and strength; thus, increased exercise and weight loss.

- Increases growth hormone; which increases energy and stamina and improves cardiac function.

This should convince you that testosterone is the hormone that protects your heart. This is not just theory. I see these benefits in my patients.

Testosterone and Bones

The most important aspect of depleted hormones in men is the loss of androgens, the hormones that build us up. Androgens are testosterone, DHEA, and growth hormone. They drop in both men and women, during andropause and menopause.

These hormones (androgens) stimulate the production of bone. Vitamin D_3 brings in calcium to strengthen bones. Vitamin K_2 (100 mcg) helps to direct the calcium to the bones, rather than to blood vessels and organs (where we don't want it). These hormones and vitamins build strong bones, the right kind of bone; unlike bisphosphonate drugs, which are commonly prescribed. Drugs such as Fosamax, Actonel, and Evista build weak bones, brittle bones. Whereas, the three androgens, D_3, and K_2 are *natural* bone builders that do an exceedingly good job. *They are the same hormones and vitamins that worked to make our bones in the first place.*

Bone loss begins around age thirty-five (for both men and women) when the androgens begin declining. Osteoporosis is almost a forgotten disease. We always assume it will happen to someone else. We also think of it as a women's disease. It happens to men, too.

The best news is that osteoporosis, and it's less severe predecessor osteopenia, are totally preventable. Bone-density scans beginning at an earlier age (forty) can accurately identify bone loss by comparing your results to the norm for your age, and comparing your current scan to any previous scans; they should start around age forty-five to fifty, and be repeated in two to five years, depending upon how good or bad the results.

Osteoporosis literally means "porous bones." It strikes 40 percent of women if they do not take hormone replacement. Men are only less vulnerable because they have a greater bone mass in their youth. However, if you plan on being around into age eighty, ninety, or a hundred, osteoporosis also may strike you.

Osteoporosis can be very debilitating, with compression fractures of the vertebrae and associated terrific back pain. Hip fractures in a "little old lady" or "little old man" can be life-ending. Also, this is a very expensive disease, which requires acute care; long-term care for those in wheel chairs and nursing homes.

Here are some facts:

- 25 million Americans suffer from osteoporosis.

- One-fifth of osteoporosis patients are men.

- By age forty, both men and women lose bone at approximately a half percent per year.

- For women, the rate of loss can increase ten-fold after menopause.

- Many women lose a third of their bone density by age sixty.

- Half of all untreated women have an osteoporotic fracture by age seventy.

- A "little old lady" with a fractured hip isn't going to live another year about 60 percent of the time.

- $10 billion is spent yearly dealing with osteoporosis.

Estrogen replacement therapy, for men as well as women, has been proven over and over again to *prevent* osteoporosis — however, men would not like the estrogen side-effects! Therefore, testosterone is also very helpful in maintaining bone mass. Men need good levels of testosterone that rival their youth. This is easily achievable. As with most things, it comes down to nutrition, exercise, and total hormonal balance.

Also, now that the medical establishment is more aware that almost everyone is deficient in vitamin D, and doctors are replacing this vitamin more routinely, we are all beginning to do better at prevention. In addition to vitamin D for bone health, everyone also needs sufficient quantities of folate, B_6, magnesium, copper, zinc, manganese, and other nutrients. Diet also is very important for bones, because bones are made of protein, which is then calcified. Weight-bearing exercise is also enormously beneficial. I cannot emphasize enough the tremendous benefit of exercise for building strong, healthy bones.

These substances contribute to bone loss:

- Sugar consumption depletes calcium and other trace minerals.

- Caffeine consumption is associated with bone loss.

- Two to three glasses of wine or cocktails daily is associated with bone loss; although alcohol in moderation seems to have little or no effect.

- Phosphorus, found in soft drinks, uses calcium and creates bone loss.

- Overdose of thyroid hormone, or hyperthyroidism, also contributes to bone loss.

Bone is actually protein that is covered with calcium, like a scaffolding; so, protein intake is critical. As a generalization, women do not eat enough protein and are protein-deficient. Too much protein is also problematic, because the body must use calcium to buffer the amino acids from the protein.

If you have osteopenia:

- Be sure to get adequate protein and calcium.

- Supplemental calcium is usually with magnesium in a 2:1 ratio. Most adults need 500-600 mg daily (you get another 500-600 mg in your diet).

- Also take vitamin D₃ (to know how much to take, get your 25-OH-Vitamin D level drawn by your doctor).

- Vitamin K also directs calcium to the bones rather than to blood vessels and organs.

- Get to a gym and do weight-bearing exercises: treadmill, stair stepper, elliptical, bike, weight lifting, Pilates. Do exercises five to six days a week. (However, not swimming; because it is not a weight-bearing activity, which is needed for bone stimulation.)

- Most important, get *total hormonal balance* with a doctor who understands bioidentical hormones: that estrogen slows the natural breakdown of bone, testosterone speeds up the natural rebuilding of bone, vitamins D and K supply the necessary calcium.

If you have osteoporosis already, do all of the above, plus the following:

- High doses of vitamin C (1,000-3,000 mg daily). This increases repair of connective tissues. It also may help to increase testosterone production and eliminate excess estrogen.

- Supplemental magnesium (200-600 mg daily "to tolerance"). Start with a magnesium citrate (200-300 mg daily the first week, double it the second week, triple it the third week, and so forth). At some point, you will develop diarrhea. Then reduce the dose to what you tolerated the previous week, and keep taking that amount. Magnesium is the most utilized mineral in the body. Therefore, it is needed for many reactions. It is also calming, and often helps with sleep.

- Manganese is also important to bone (5-20 mg daily). Most of us are deficient, because it is not in our foods with the advent of "modern" farming techniques that strip the soil of minerals.

- Folate, B_6, and B_{12} help to prevent a buildup of the amino acid homocysteine; which, when elevated, triples the risk of osteoporosis, heart disease, and dementia. These three vitamins are in "B Complex," which is especially recommended if you have joint pain or osteoporosis.

- Boron is a trace mineral needed in bone formation (1-3 mg daily). It enhances the production of compounds related to bone health; including estrogen, testosterone, DHEA, and vitamin D.

Testosterone and Prostate Health

Abraham Morgentaler, M.D.'s book *Testosterone for Life* has reversed what has been "common knowledge" for doctors for decades. He has shown clearly that testosterone has been unfairly accused of causing prostate cancer. In fact, the reverse is true.

Testosterone therapy is safe for the prostate gland. In fact, of concern now is the growing evidence that low testosterone is a risk *for* prostate cancer! Here is a short synopsis of the prostate story.

The original work showing that testosterone was linked to an increased risk of prostate cancer was done by Nobel Prize winners. Charles Huggins was a urologist at the University of Chicago. He was interested in a condition of prostatic enlargement, called benign prostatic hypertrophy (BPH); a condition that causes frequent and urgent urination, and sometimes obstructs the urethra. Huggins was doing experiments on BPH in dogs. He noted that castration relieved the problem; he also noted that prostate cancers shrank with the castration of the dogs.

So, next, Huggins applied the dog studies to humans. He either castrated the men, or chemically castrated them by using estrogen. In the 1940s and early 1950s, this was commonly done to men who had prostate cancer or BPH; and they did have to give their consent. Huggins found that the blood test acid *phosphatase* was high in men who had prostate cancer; however, the test normalized with lowering testosterone levels. The study's finding was that *lowering* testosterone causes a prostate cancer to *shrink.* This report of prostate cancer being dependent on testosterone levels was very important, because in the 1940s there was no other known treatment for prostate cancer. Thus, lowering testosterone became the main treatment for this advanced disease . . . and it has been the standard of care, until recently.

Lowering testosterone methods have changed from estrogen or castration, to medications like Lupron developed in the 1980s. Huggins received a Nobel Prize for his work on prostate cancer and testosterone levels; his work was not seriously questioned until very recently.

Along came Dr. Morgentaler, who did his urology training at the famed Harvard Program. He learned the common thoughts regarding testosterone and prostate cancer. When he started his own practice, primarily male infertility and sexual problems, he began diagnosing and treating men who had low testosterone.

This was not common at the time, so a former professor of Morgentaler's advised him that he shouldn't be doing these treatments, at least not without first doing prostate biopsies, to be sure he wasn't adding "fuel to the fire" of prostate cancer. This advice upset the young Morgentaler; nevertheless, he did perform the prostate biopsies, on his own patients who had low testosterone. Interestingly, by digital rectal exam (DRG), these men had *normal* prostate exams and *normal* prostate-specific antigen (PSA) blood tests. At the time, DRG and PSA were thought to be the best way to detect prostate cancer, and prostate cancer certainly was not linked to low testosterone. Surprisingly, of these normally low-risk men, six of the thirty-three had cancer, an abnormally high cancer rate.

Dr. Morgentaler reported his findings at a national urology meeting. The news wasn't received well, because it flew in the face of what had been "known" for decades. He continued on, however. He biopsied an additional group of men, 200 patients; and the 14 percent cancer rate remained the same. He submitted his new data to the prestigious *Journal of the American Medical Association* (*JAMA*, 1996). At that time, Morgentaler's reported rate of cancer (14%) was considered exceedingly high, especially since this was a "low risk" group of men. This was the first evidence that standard assumptions about testosterone and prostate cancer might be in error.

If we examine the natural progression of prostate cancer, we find that young men in their twenties (when one's testosterone level is at its maximum), do not have prostate cancer. From autopsies of young men, we know that a significant percentage of young men harbor microscopic cancers. By comparison, prostate cancer increases as men age . . . and their testosterone level falls.

This observation is opposite of the prevailing theory, even today: that low testosterone is protective against prostate cancer. Physicians still commonly withhold testosterone treatment from men who have known low testosterone, because of the "old" *disproven* fear that it will cause prostate cancer. *It will not.*

In Morgentaler's review of literature on prostate cancer risk for men receiving testosterone therapy, he found only small studies showing a prostate cancer rate (slighty > 1%) less than the detection rate found in general screenings of men. Of long-term studies looking at testosterone levels in large groups of men, following these groups to see who developed prostate cancer over twenty years, there was *no* association between testosterone levels and the risk of developing prostate cancer. In a thorough review of the literature, Dr. Morgentaler did *not* find a single study showing high testosterone associated with increased risk of prostate cancer!

His research next led him to the basement of the Harvard library where he found the original 1941 article by Huggins and co-investigator, Clarence Hodges; who had studied only three men and had published the results from only two men. One of those two men already had been castrated, meaning the study was comprised of only *one* man! Dr. Huggins had based his conclusion, that testosterone injections cause "enhanced growth" of prostate cancer, on a single man! Plus, he used the acid phosphatase test that has since been *abandoned* because it has been found to be too erratic. Dr.

Morgentaler wrote, "Dr. Huggin's assertion that higher testosterone caused greater growth of prostate cancer, repeated for so long and accepted as gospel, was based on almost nothing at all!"

There is a developing paradox. We've known for decades that lowering testosterone levels causes a positive result (the prostate shrinks) and raising testosterone levels causes it to grow. Although the second part is now very doubtful, the first part is definitely true.

All of the studies on testosterone therapy resulting in rapid growth of prostate cancer, occurred in men who already had extremely low testosterone levels due to castration or estrogen therapy. There is *no* evidence that changes in testosterone level matters at all when we start with testosterone levels that are not in the castrate range.

In 2006, Dr. Leonard Marks et al. published an article titled "Effect of Testosterone Replacement Therapy on Prostate Tissue in Men with Late-onset Hypogonadism: A randomized controlled trial" (*JAMA*), which resolved the issue. They showed that in the testosterone (T) treatment group's blood concentration of T and dehydrotestosterone (DHT) rose substantially, as they should. However, the concentration of T and DHT in the prostate itself remained constant, and was similar to the placebo group. Biomarkers of prostate stimulation did not change with testosterone treatment.

This showed that raising testosterone levels in the blood stream does *not* change levels in the prostate. At some point, the prostate becomes saturated, so the testosterone level does not rise. So, the paradox is resolved!

At very low levels of testosterone, as in the castrate range, the prostate is very sensitive to changes in testosterone levels. *Therefore, very low levels of testosterone will allow a prostate to* **shrink.**

Likewise, adding testosterone back will stimulate a prostate to grow. Once the saturation with testosterone has been exceeded (>50ng/dl), adding more will have little further effect. The blood level to achieve saturation is quite low (>50ng/dl). The target for testosterone therapy is 700-900 ng/dl. At castrate levels (<50ng/dl) the prostate is sensitive to changes in the testosterone level. However, even men with very low testosterone are in the range of 200-300 ng/dl. Anything above 50ng/dl creates no change in prostate testosterone level. So, almost all men will not have a change in the prostate level of testosterone when their blood level is raised through testosterone supplementation.

Also, treating men with low testosterone does not affect the prostate. However, it does bring nice changes for the individual: more energy, clearer thinking, less fat, better sleep, and better sexual function.

Following this line of reasoning, I have *no concern* that giving a man testosterone supplementation will promote or initiate a prostate cancer. Rather, I *am* concerned that men with *low* testosterone (most men over age fifty) are at an *increased* risk.

Dr. Rhoden and Dr. Morgentaler published another study in 2006 in the *International Journal of Impotence Research;* showing in 345 men that "the degree of testosterone deficiency correlated with the degree of cancer risk. Men whose testosterone levels were in the bottom third of the group were twice as likely to have cancer diagnosed on biopsy as men in the upper third. This finding adds to the concern that low T is a risk factor for prostate cancer." *Other studies are also now telling us that low testosterone is associated with more aggressive tumors.*

In summary, Dr. Morgentaler has taught us that men who already have metastatic prostate cancer and have been given treatment that dropped their blood level of testosterone to near zero, starting treatment of testosterone (or stopping treatment that lowered their testosterone to near zero) might increase the risk that residual cancer will again start to grow.

However, while a *low* blood level of testosterone does not protect against prostate cancer and, indeed, may increase the risk:

- A *high* blood level of testosterone does not increase the risk and may, in fact, protect against prostate cancer. Just as significant, according to Morgentaler:

- Testosterone replenishment does *not* increase the risk of prostate cancer, even among men already at high risk for it.

Risks of Testosterone Replacement in Men

As long as one is not overdosed, the risks are minimal. Some men worry that they might get cancer or heart disease from taking testosterone supplementation. Actually, the opposite is true, as shown above. Not taking testosterone, when deficient, can result in these diseases. In studies of men who previously had prostate cancer, compared to those who did not, the group with the lowest testosterone levels had more cancer. In studies of men with heart disease, the group of men with lower testosterone levels had more heart attacks. *So, testosterone is disease preventing.*

Known possible risks are testicular atrophy and decreased sperm count; however, with appropriate doses, these risks are very low.

Concerned about prostate cancer? Although you will find several under-informed doctors (the majority) who believe that testosterone supplementation increases a man's risk of developing prostate cancer, the reverse is true. Men with low testosterone levels are more likely to develop prostate cancer than men who have a normal or even slightly high level. The bigger culprit for men is estrogen (which naturally rises with age).

To avoid prostate cancer:

- Eat lots of fruits and vegetables, especially cruciferous vegetables (broccoli, Brussel sprouts, cauliflower, cabbage, kale, mustard greens).

- Reduce stress and get adequate sleep (7-8 hours).

- Exercise regularly.

- Keep weight normal.

- Supplement vitamin D$_3$ to normal levels (60-80) by blood tests. This usually means taking a vitamin D$_3$ pill containing 2,000 to 4,000 units daily. Get a blood test to see if you are deficient. I have found that 98 percent of my patients were deficient.

- Keep your testosterone level in the appropriate range (700-900 mg/dl).

Forms Available of Testosterone Replacement

Testosterone is easy to measure with a blood test. We often start with a transdermal cream. Some men do well with the cream (or a lozenge or troche). The negative of the cream for men is that it can increase the risk of converting testosterone into DHT. There are skin patches for men, but they frequently cause irritation and often provide an inadequate dose. Therefore, the most recommended way for men to replace testosterone loss is by injection, and the best form of that is testosterone cypionate in a multi-dose vial. It's a small quantity, so it's easy to administer. The injections are usually given twice weekly.

Another possibility for treatment is the use of human chorionic gonadotropin (HCG). This is the hormone measured in a pregnancy test; it's made by placenta. HCG is very close in structure to luetinizing hormone (LH), which stimulates the production of testosterone by the testes. In this situation, the body misreads HCG enough so that testosterone production is promoted. This works in younger men, and recently andropausal men. After a few years of this treatment, or in most older men, the testes fail to respond to the HCG stimulus and the patient then needs to switch to testosterone cypionate injections twice weekly.

Forms of Andropause

Testosterone production depends upon an area of the brain called the hypothalamus. This is where the brain monitors levels of the various hormones, including testosterone. When testosterone is low, the hypothalamus sends a message to the pituitary gland (a part of the brain) via the gonadotropin releasing hormone (GnRH), which stimulates the pituitary to respond by secreting the lutenizing hormone (LH) and the follicle stimulating hormone (FSH). LH then goes to the testicles, where it stimulates the Leydig cells to manufacture more testosterone. In this way, the brain monitors the hormone levels and stimulates production of needed hormones to maintain homeostasis. (This is analogous to estrogen production in women, also controlled by the pituitary.)

One form of andropause happens when the hypothalamus or pituitary is not working properly; therefore, the stimulus to make testosterone does not go out, or not in a timely fashion.

In the case of primary hypogonadism, the Leydig cells lose their natural ability to respond to the pituitary stimulus; the testosterone levels, therefore, are low. In the case of secondary hypogonadism, there is a pituitary failure and the hormones LH and FSH are not made. Even though the testicles might be in good working order, they have no stimulus to make testosterone; therefore, the testosterone production lowers, and the testosterone levels in the blood stream are low.

In my experience, *secondary hypogandism* is a more common cause of low testosterone in middle-aged men. However, the most *significant* form of andropause is not caused by a deficiency of testosterone, either primary or secondary; rather, by a more complex hormone disorder. In fact, the measurement of the testosterone levels could be normal.

Follow Ups on Testosterone Supplementation

It is very important to follow up with men who have initiated testosterone therapy. Your doctor needs to follow the DHT (dehydrotestosterone) and estradiol levels, as well as the testosterone and free testosterone levels. We also watch the PSA (prostate specific antigen) level to make sure it doesn't change during testosterone supplementation.

Some men's bodies convert testosterone into DHT (dehydrotestosterone), which happens from an enzyme (5 alpha reductase) that is rich in the hair follicles. The significance of DHT increase is debated, however. It used to be thought that this caused an increased risk of prostate cancer; yet, with Morgentaler's work, that myth was dispelled. DHT might be, however, associated with increased male pattern baldness.

As men age, our bodies also tend to convert more and more testosterone into estrogen. In fact, some sixty-year-old men have higher estrogen levels than their wives! Women also have some testosterone in their bodies. It is the quantities of these hormones that vastly differs between the genders.

Nature intended for men to have *some* estrogen, so this conversion process is actually *necessary* for men's health. Men's bodies need to make *some* estrogen for our estrogen-sensitive tissues — like the brain! Estrogen also influences our natural sexual functions through its effects upon our brain chemistry. Dr. Eugene Shippen, author of *The Testosterone Syndrome,* wrote, "Too little estrogen will neuter a man just as effectively as too little testosterone." This is rare, but can happen. Shippen pointed out, "The window of optimum effectiveness in the male body is very small."

Men's bodies convert testosterone into *some* amount of estrogen (estradiol) through the enzyme aromatase. Yet the estrogen level in men's bodies does need to be controlled and kept at normal low levels. So, we can't have no estrogen, and we can't have too much. By middle age, many men have a testosterone-to-estrogen ratio that is out of balance. So, it is especially important to monitor estrogen in men who are taking testosterone supplementation, because elevated estrogen can cause an increase in clotting factors and a restriction in the caliber of the coronary arteries, increasing the risk of heart attack and/or developing prostate cancer.

Too much estrogen in men is also an "off" switch. High estrogen not only affects a man's sexuality but has other negative metabolic effects, like brain fog. We lose energy and muscle tone, put on fat, lose our competitive spirit — and may even grow "man boobs" (gynecomastia). High estrogen in men is further exacerbated by a poor diet, obesity, zinc deficiency, too much alcohol, drugs, and/or illness. In particular, fat increases estrogen production — a good reason to watch the diet!

In addition to watching the DHT and estradiol levels, your doctor also follows general health markers: cholesterol; HgbA1c (tells us the average blood sugar over the past two months); hsCRP (highly sensitive C Reactive Protein, tells us the level of inflammation in the body); homocysteine (an amino acid that, if elevated, is associated with a three times greater risk of heart disease, osteoporosis, dementia); and the vitamins D_3 and B_{12}.

Perhaps the most important aspect of checking and re-checking during your testosterone therapy is to titrate the testosterone levels to achieve the optimal levels for your individual blood stream.

With testosterone replacement therapy, it is important to follow-up every two to three months until the correct dosage is achieved; then every four to six months. Your doctor needs to recheck:

- Both Total testosterone and Free testosterone levels, to verify the optimal balance.

- PSA, to assure the absence of prostate cancer.

- Estradiol, to assure that testosterone is not inappropriately converting into unwanted estrogen (which some men do with or without testosterone treatment, and this can be controlled).

- DHT (dihydrotestosterone), to verify that testosterone is not converting inappropriately into this more potent form of testosterone that is associated with prostate enlargement and hair loss). (Men's bodies also can make this conversion with or without testosterone treatment; it also can be controlled.)

- Vitamin D_3, to maintain the optimal level for your body.

Excess Testosterone in Men

Excess testosterone is rarely seen in men, except maybe in body builders or athletes; and then it is usually self administered, illegally. Men can develop what is referred to as "roid rage." Simply stated, that is being overly aggressive, having quick anger.

Excess testosterone has negative effects upon one's physiology: increased cholesterol, triglycerides and LDL, decreased HDL (the "good cholesterol"); and increased risk of heart disease, erectile dysfunction, diminished sperm count and infertility.

Many physicians believe that excess testosterone is related to hair loss and prostate cancer. Actually, neither of these is true.

Do Men Need Progesterone?

Most men do not. It is rarely used for lowering estradiol in the body. I do not support using progesterone in men, because I think it kills libido in men; and prolonged usage may be associated with an increased risk of diabetes.

DHEA

Another hormone important for men is dihydroepiandosterone acetate, or DHEA, which is a good stimulator of the immune system. This is another androgen, like testosterone. It helps to lower cancer risk and diminish the risk of colds and flu. Some people call DHEA the "feel good hormone," because it enhances mood and a sense of well-being. It assists with weight loss; enhances libido (when combined with testosterone) and possibly fertility. It also protects brain, bones, and breast.

DHEA (dihydroepiandosterone acetate) comes mostly from the adrenal glands. Commonly, as testosterone wanes during andropause, DHEA also drops. It declines with age, as well as with adrenal burnout. We also monitor the levels of DHEA (sulfated form, DHEAS). Being the most abundant hormone in the body, it is important to balance it.

The most common form of DHEA is in pill form at 25-50 mg, easy to find over-the-counter. It can be compounded by a pharmacist into a cream or lozenge.

The risks for men are very few. Acne or oily skin may occur, if overdosed. If this happens, the dose may be reduced. For example, cut back to 10 mg until the acne goes away. Then increase the dose again. Some men don't tolerate any dose at all. Sometimes you might have to switch to 7-keto DHEA, although this is rare for men.

So, what happened to me? you might ask.

We all get older. We think this getting old thing is steady, downhill, and irreversible. *Simply — that is no longer true.* You can control, to some degree, the aging process: by taking care of yourself with good nutritional choices, consistent exercise, stress management, adequate sleep, and avoiding toxins like caffeine, sugar, alcohol, and tobacco.

What most men have missed up until now is *invigorating* hormone replacement. For a healthy physiology, men must address the issue of optimal levels of hormones in their bodies; because hormones affect muscles, bones, skin, energy, mood, and sexual performance. It's easier to heal and fight off infection. We sleep better and have more energy.

You may have tried various diets to lose weight, gone faithfully to a gym, perhaps even tried meditating. These are all reasonable things to do. However, reversing the aging process goes beyond these usual methods.

The key factor is *metabolism*. To regain our optimal metabolism, we men must restore our *optimal* hormonal levels. This is how we regain our normal weight and normal energy, a sharp mind, the vigor to compete again, and restore sexual performance and a loving relationship.

It's odd that we men refer to our hormones as sex hormones — when they do so much more! We all see the changes in our vision as we go to "readers." However, as we age, we are also losing brain power and memory, lung capacity, kidney function, cardiac function, bone strength, and digestive function.

Think, for a moment, about sagging skin and relate that to your bowel. Have you considered what your *insides* look like? It's a mirror image. We can see what is going on with our skin as it wrinkles, sags, loses elasticity. If our outside is sagging, imagine what our insides are like. If our bowel looks like and functions like our skin, we could be in deep trouble. The bowel is where 70 percent of our immune system resides, and where we digest and absorb food for energy, strength, normal functioning, and cellular repairs.

We are only as young as our most diseased part. To avoid, or at least put off, the diseases of aging, and restore vigor: Commit to good nutrition, consistent exercise, stress management, adequate sleep, detoxifying and cleaning up toxic habits (e.g., smoking, drinking, too much sugar, too much caffeine) — and restore your optimal hormonal levels.

Health is a choice! You *can* feel younger and more vital! You *can* enhance your outward appearance and inner health. You can again have an enjoyable life, a more vigorous life. Go back and re-read the information on inflammation, oxidation, glycation, poor methylation, detoxification, and thrombosis. These are the faulty processes that take the body down, that lead to disease, that *can* be reined in. You can slow down or minimize your risk of heart disease, diabetes, hypertension, cancer, joint disease (e.g., arthritis), dementia. The single-most important factor is restoring diminished hormonal levels.

In our youth, we were ready to play ball, climb mountains, ski steep terrain, and conquer the neighborhood, city, state. That is the vigor of youth. *That* is what hormones do. They refuel our youth!

Treating, and beating, andropause is not difficult — and the changes in how you feel and look are enormous!

Conclusion

How Do You Know What's Making You Feel the Way You Do?

Y ou don't know. That is why you go to a professional who has spent years learning how to approach and solve these complicated problems.

This is not a self-help book. The information presented here is to try to give you some ideas about what you can do for yourself . . . and what kinds of things a physician might do to help you.

How do you know what's making you sick, when symptoms are similar for many causes? One post-menopausal woman proposed a number of questions to me regarding common chronic symptoms as well as new ones.

What is the underlying cause of changes in your sleep patterns? Is it just that you aren't getting a good night's sleep? Is something causing it?

I have been surprised by the number of people who do not sleep well. Many times, it is the lack of hormones associated with menopause or andropause.

- *Progesterone,* for example, is very calming and helps women sleep.

- Lack of *estrogen* is upsetting enough for many women that they don't sleep well until they get their hormones balanced.

- *Melatonin* is a brain hormone that is often lacking. One can get melatonin over-the-counter in health-food stores and compounding pharmacies. Anywhere from 1 mg to 18 mgs may be necessary.

- Sometimes people need *magnesium* supplementation. Magnesium is used in more chemical reactions than any other mineral, and most of us are deficient. Take magnesium "to tolerance." Get magnesium citrate or glycinate, 100 mg to 300 mg. The first week, take one daily. The second week, two daily. The third week, three daily. Keep increasing the dose in this way. At some point, you will get diarrhea. When that happens, simply cut back the dose to the one you previously took and tolerated. This will be your tolerance level. Magnesium is good for many things, like sleep, blood-pressure control, and muscle function.

Is your extreme fatigue (which has haunted you for as many decades as you can remember and is almost crippling at times) the result of adrenal exhaustion, osteoporosis, vitamin D insufficiency, stress-stress-stress (and you already meditate and do all those "calming" things), insufficient exercise (light walking), chronic fatigue syndrome (not traditionally recognized diagnosis); and/or chronic lifelong headaches, allergies, and sinusitis (often not recognized as a serious component and disease)?

This list makes me think of adrenal exhaustion. Adrenal exhaustion makes you feel terrible, with no energy. It is caused by stress, over-exercise, inadequate nutrition, toxins, and maybe from some vitamin deficiencies piling on. With adrenal exhaustion, one also has lowered immunity to colds, flu, and sinus infection. With adrenal exhaustion, one feels too poorly to exercise and cannot make enough cortisol to support exercise anyway; at the depth of adrenal exhaustion, exercise only makes matters worse. So it is very important to have this diagnosed, because exercising is necessary for optimal well-being and good health overall. No excuses! If you do have adrenal exhaustion, remedy it, so that you can live a full and abundant life.

If you just had your first-ever bone-density scan at age sixty-five and learn that you have osteoporosis (when you should have started getting scans at age forty), what can you do about it now? Can it be reversed?

Absolutely. The most effective way to reverse any kind of bone loss is fitting in everything taught in this book. In particular:

- *Estrogen* slows the rate of bone degradation.

- *Testosterone* supplementation speeds up the rebuilding of bone.

- *Vitamin D* helps to promote the absorption of calcium into the body.

- *Vitamin K* helps to direct the calcium into the bones, rather than other tissues where calcium may not belong.

- *Weight-bearing exercise* stimulates extra bone growth.

- Abundant *protein* intake is necessary because the basic bone structure is comprised of protein. Unfortunately, many women consume inadequate amounts of protein in their diets.

How much estrogen supplementation do you need to rebuild the bone density, and how long will it take?

As stated above, *estrogen* will help. It also helps mood and the general feeling of well-being. A minimum of 50 ng/ml of estradiol in the blood stream provides adequate assistance for bone stability. Many big pharmaceutical companies' estrogen products do not achieve estrogen levels even close to 50 ng/ml, and most OB/Gyns don't know the difference. This is another reason to find a doctor who specializes in Age Management Medicine.

Bones change very slowly. To see a change in bone density level, wait two years to recheck with the bone densitometry test.

It is also essential to have adequate levels of vitamin D. The levels need to be in the range of 60 to 80 to obtain the *optimal* help from the vitamin D supplement.

Are deficiencies the cause of these diseases?

I would not say all, but it is the cause of many problems. We've stated that everyone needs adequate and good nutrition, with good vitamin and mineral support. Everyone also needs consistent exercise and total hormonal balance. Deficiency in any of these things does lead to increased risk of diseases.

For additional very significant statistics and data on addressing osteoporosis and osteopenia, please see the comprehensive discussion in the Men's Manual in the section titled "Testosterone and Bones." Bone disease affects both women and men.

How can you know the origin of sudden high blood pressure, when you've never had it before?

In most people, the cause of high blood pressure is unknown (called idiopathic) and requires the diagnosis of a physician. There are some medical causes of high blood pressure, like kidney disease. The important thing is that it be identified and treated. Sometimes high blood pressure can be modified downward with magnesium, potassium, and/or arginine. Oftentimes, people need antihypertensive medications.

How can you know the cause of rapid heartbeat, inner trembling, constant chronic headaches, that are especially noticeable upon waking.

These, too, require the help of a qualified physician. Possibly an endocrinologist, internist, or OB/Gyn. You need a physician who has studied *beyond* internship and residency. This could be a physician knowledgeable about Functional Medicine, Alternative Medicine, or Holistic Medicine. Knowledge of hormones would be very helpful as well. In a city the size of Denver (2 million people), for example, there are only a handful of physicians who would qualify.

When symptoms can be caused by any number of origins, and causes can overlap, how can you identify the most likely culprit? How can you get well? Where do you begin to solve your health puzzle?

An answer to this question is beyond the scope of this book. This is what we learn in years of medical school. First, you need a diagnosis. Once the root problem has been identified, then the doctor can offer appropriate solutions. Lab testing reveals a lot, so I recommend a full spectrum of blood tests and analyses, combined with a thorough medical history of symptoms and treatments.

Fundamental Medicine teaches us to take a thorough medical history, look over what already has been done, do a physical examination, then do appropriate testing; whether that is x-ray, ultrasound, blood testing, urine testing, possibly saliva testing, or other. Hopefully, the tests given will reveal the health challenge that is causing the symptoms or malady. Playing detective is part of it. Wisdom and intuition are also key components to identifying the appropriate test that will identify the underlying cause of symptoms and help to discern the right solution.

The best course of treatment is dictated by the diagnosis. Getting a good history from the patient often gives insight. Sometimes there are treatment choices; sometimes there aren't. Different people require different testing. There is generally a lot of overlap in the tests that I do.

The goal is to bring all of the information together to determine which physiological system (e.g., immune, detoxification, digestion, endocrine, neurologic, energy production) is needing the most help. Again, it requires a good history, an examination, and some lab work.

Putting it all together can be challenging. Allowing enough time when you are sick, and tired of being sick, takes a doctor with understanding and patience. When a doctor can determine the worst problem and the system most in need of treatment, things begin to get better. As one system is restored, the miraculous body oftentimes then can heal the other weakened systems.

How do you know what kind of doctor(s) to see? Where can you go for the real answers? The internet? Self-help books by doctors? The yellow pages?

Finding a knowledgeable doctor to help with these kinds of problems is difficult. Doctors who enjoy this type of work are trying to get their names out there; such as through speaking, classes and workshops, writing books, and providing websites.

These websites are a helpful resource: the American Association of Anti-Aging Medicine, www.worldhealth.net; the Institute of Functional Medicine, www.functionalmedicine.org; Age Management Medicine Group, www.AgeMed.org; www.SuzanneSomers.com; www.LifeExtension.com. The difficulty with some online directories is that physicians who do only cosmetic procedures are listed along with those who focus on hormones and nutrition. I believe that physicians listed in these directories are cutting-edge, wise physicians.

Where do you get the help you really need? How can you tell if that is the right approach for your body, history, and symptoms? How do you convince your doctor or PCP that your symptoms are not due to merely emotional stress or tension, but feel physiological in origin?

Same answers as above. You have to find someone like me who is interested in these kinds of health challenges. I think most people can tell when they "click" with their doctor. Check out the choices by websites. Check Google to see what might come up on a certain doctor.

You can feel yourself struggling to find your health answers. You have tried everything you can to find the solutions. Still, you feel really lousy and there seems to be no hope. Is there hope? If so, how and where do you find it?

Yes, there is hope. Find the right doctor. (See above.)

Dr. Ray D. Strand, author of *What Your Doctor Doesn't Know About Nutritional Medicine,* reminds us that to regain our health, we need nutritional medicine and cellular nutrition. I agree. The strategies I have outlined in this book are a solid foundation for better health. When you follow the Age Management plan provided here, you *will* feel and look better. It *is* possible.

The secret to great health is really pretty simple. The cornerstones of good health are: adequate and reasonable nutrition, optimal supplements, adequate and enjoyable exercise, uninterrupted hours of sleep (adults 7 to 9), stress management, and total hormonal balance.

Choose good organic foods. Follow the Glycemic Index. Avoid saturated and trans fats. Don't worry about Omega 3 (fish and flax seeds) and Omega 9 fats (nuts, avocados); they're good for you! Supplement your diet with vitamins and minerals, to counteract whatever might be ailing you, or to correct deficiencies.

I recommend the following supplements for most everybody, though some individuals may need more depending upon their circumstances:

- Omega 3 fish oil, purified (3,000 mg of DHA plus EPA)

- Probiotics daily

- Good multivitamin/multimineral (e.g., Nutrilite's Double X)

- Vitamin D_3 (check your level) with vitamin K 100 mcg

- Calcium/magnesium citrate, 600 mg/300 mg daily

- An antioxidant — many, many choices

   - Vitamin C (1,000-2,000 mg daily)

   - Mixed vitamin E (800 units daily)

   - Mixed carotenes (15,000-25,000 units daily)

- N-acetyl cysteine (600 mg daily)

- Women: DIM 300 mg daily (di-indole methane)

- Men: Saw palmetto, with nettle root, daily.

To improve your strength, stamina, flexibility and endurance: exercise, consistently. Manage your stress in a way that is enjoyable to you, get plenty of good sleep, achieve your *optimal* levels of hormonal restoration — *and* you will create a positive, uplifting, and joyful attitude toward life!

Regarding hormone replacement therapy, different conclusions are reached by different doctors, depending upon their knowledge and research. My goal is your optimal health so you can enjoy your life to the fullest.

I am convinced that the principles outlined in this book will move everyone toward better health. I believe we all can be healthier, possibly even extend our years, by replenishing our body's nutrition, supplements, exercise, sleep, and hormonal needs. We can live full of energy and joy — while pursuing our passions and helping others.

The one area where we do have some control in life is our health. Functional and Age Management doctors aim for the stars in our care of the human body and your whole being. We are ready to help you feel like yourself again — to feel wonderful!

Appendices

Appendix

Glycemic Index

What Is the Glycemic Index?

The Glycemic Index (GI) is one the best tools for fat loss. It measures how quickly foods breakdown into sugar in the bloodstream. High glycemic foods turn into blood sugar very quickly. Starchy foods, like potatoes, are a good example. Potatoes have such a high GI rating that it's almost the same as eating table sugar.

The GI tells you how fast foods spike your blood sugar (but won't tell you how much carbohydrate per serving you're getting). That's where the Glycemic Load is a great help.

What is the Glycemic Load (GL)?

The Glycemic Load measures the amount of *carbohydrate* in each serving of food. When considering the Glycemic Load also consider the Glycemic Index. Ideally, you want them both to be low. *Glycemic Index* choices should be foods *less than* 47.

Good Choice:

Foods with a *glycemic load* under 10.

These foods should be your first choice for carbs.

Moderate Choice:

Foods that fall between 10 and 20 on the glycemic load scale.

They have a reasonable affect on your blood sugar.

Poor Choice:

Foods with a glycemic load above 20.

These will cause blood sugar and insulin spikes.

Sparingly eat foods with a glycemic load of 20.

Food	Glycemic Index	Serving Size (g)	Glycemic Load
CANDY/SWEETS			
Honey	87	2 Tbs	17.9
Jelly Beans	78	1 oz	22
Snickers Bar	68	60g (1/2 bar)	23
Table Sugar	68	2 Tsp	7
Strawberry Jam	51	2 Tbs	10.1

Peanut M&M's	33	30 g (1 oz)	5.6
Dove Dark Chocolate Bar	23	37g (1 oz)	4.4
BAKED GOODS & CEREALS			
Corn Bread	110	60g (1 piece)	30.8
French Bread	95	64g (1 slice)	29.5
Corn Flakes	92	28g (1 cup)	21.1
Corn Chex	83	30g (1 cup)	20.8
Rice Krispies	82	33g (1.25 cup)	23
Corn Pops	80	31g (1 cup)	22.4
Donut, large glazed	76	75g (1 donut)	24.3
Waffle, homemade	76	75g (1 waffle)	18.7
Grape Nuts	75	58g (1/2 cup)	31.5
Bran Flakes	74	29g (3/4 cup)	13.3
Graham Cracker	74	14g (2 sqrs)	8.1
Cheerios	74	30g (1 cup)	13.3
Kaiser Roll	73	57g (1 roll)	21.2

Bagel	72	89g (1/4 in.)	33
Corn Tortilla	70	24g (1 tortilla)	7.7
Melba Toast	70	12g (4 rounds)	5.6
Wheat Bread	70	28g (1 slice)	7.7
White Bread	70	25g (1 slice)	8.4
Kellogg's Special K	69	31g (1 cup)	14.5
Taco Shell	68	13g (1 med)	4.8
Angel Food Cake	67	28g (1 slice)	10.7
Croissant, Butter	67	57g (1 med)	17.5
Muselix	66	55g (2/3 cup)	23.8
Oatmeal, instant	65	234g (1 cup)	13.7
Rye Bread, 100% whole	65	32g (1 slice)	8.5
Rye Krisp Crackers	65	25 (1 wafer)	11.1
Raisin Bran	61	61g (1 cup)	24.4
Bran Muffin	60	113g (1 med)	30
Blueberry Muffin	59	113g (1 med)	30
Oatmeal	58	117g (1/2 cup)	6.4
Whole Wheat Pita	57	64g (1 pita)	17

Oatmeal Cookie	55	18g (1 large)	6
Popcorn	55	8g (1 cup)	2.8
Pound cake, Sara Lee	54	30g (1 piece)	8.1
Vanilla Cake and Vanilla Frosting	42	64g (1 slice)	16
Pumpernickel Bread	41	26g (1slice)	4.5
Chocolate Cake and Chocolate Frosting	38	64g (1 slice)	12.5
BEVERAGES			
Gatorade Powder	78	16g (.75 scoop)	11.7
Cranberry Juice Cocktail	68	253g (1 cup)	24.5
Cola, Carbonated	63	370g (12oz can)	25.2
Orange Juice	57	249g (1 cup)	14.25
Hot Chocolate Mix	51	28g (1 packet)	11.7
Grapefruit Juice, sweetened	48	250g (1 cup)	13.4
Pineapple Juice	46	250g (1 cup)	14.7
Soy Milk	44	245g (1 cup)	4

Apple Juice	41	248g (1 cup)	11.9
Tomato Juice	38	243g (1 cup)	3.4
LEGUMES			
Baked Beans	48	253g (1 cup)	18.2
Pinto Beans	39	171g (1 cup)	11.7
Lima Beans	31	241g (1 cup)	7.4
Chickpeas, boiled	31	240g (1 cup)	13.3
Lentils	29	198g (1 cup)	7
Kidney Beans	27	256g (1 cup)	7
Soy Beans	20	172g (1 cup)	1.4
Peanuts	13	146g (1 cup)	1.6
VEGETABLES			
Potato	104	213g (1 med)	36.4
Parsnip	97	78g (1/2 cup)	11.6
Carrot, raw	92	15g (1 large)	1
Beets, canned	64	246g (1/2 cup)	9.6
Corn Yellow	55	166g (1 cup)	61.5
Sweet Potato	54	133g (1 cup)	12.4

Yam	51	136g (1 cup)	16.8
Peas, frozen	48	72g (1/2 cup)	3.4
Tomato	38	123g (1 med)	1.5
Broccoli, cooked	0	78g (1/2 cup)	0
Cabbage, cooked	0	75g (1/2 cup)	0
Celery, raw	0	62g (1 stalk)	0
Cauliflower	0	100g (1 cup)	0
Green Beans	0	135g (1 cup)	0
Mushrooms	0	70g (1 cup)	0
Spinach	0	30g (1 cup)	0
FRUIT			
Watermelon	72	152g (1 cup)	7.2
Pineapple, raw	66	155g (1 cup)	11.9
Cantaloupe	65	177g (1 cup)	7.8
Apricot, canned in light syrup	64	253g (1 cup)	24.3
Raisins	64	43g (small box)	20.5
Papaya	60	140g (1 cup)	6.6

Peaches, canned, heavy syrup	58	262g (1 cup)	28.4
Kiwi, with skin	58	76g (1 fruit)	5.2
Fruit Cocktail, drained	55	214g (1 cup)	19.8
Peaches, canned, light syrup	52	251g (1 cup)	17.7
Banana	51	118g (1 med)	12.2
Mango	51	165g (1 cup)	12.8
Orange	48	140g (1 fruit)	7.2
Pears, canned in pear juice	44	248g (1 cup)	12.3
Grapes	43	92g (1 cup)	6.5
Strawberries	40	152g (1 cup)	3.6
Apple, with skin	39	138g (1 med)	6.2
Pear	33	166g (1 med)	6.9
Apricot, dried	32	130g (1 cup)	23
Prunes	29	132g (1 cup)	34.2
Peach	28	98g (1 med)	2.2

Grapefruit	25	123g (1/2 fruit)	2.8
Plum	24	66g (1 fruit)	1.7
Sweet Cherries, raw	22	117g (1 cup)	3.7
NUTS			
Cashews	22		
Almonds	0		
Hazelnuts	0		
Macadamia	0		
Pecans	0		
Walnuts	0		
DAIRY			
Ice Cream, lower fat	47	76g (1/2 cup)	9.4
Pudding	44	100g (1/2 cup)	8.4
Milk, whole	40	244g (1 cup)	4.4
Ice Cream	38	72g (1/2 cup)	6
Yogurt, plain	36	245g (1 cup)	6.1
MEAT/PROTEIN			
Beef	0		

Chicken	0		
Eggs	0		
Fish	0		
Lamb	0		
Pork	0		
Veal	0		
Deer-Venison	0		
Elk	0		
Buffalo	0		
Rabbit	0		
Duck	0		
Ostrich	0		
Shellfish	0		
Lobster	0		
Turkey	0		
Ham	0		

Tips for Fat Busting Meals

Avoid:

- Grains, including corn and rice
- Potatoes and other white foods; like white rice, sugar, salt
- Processed foods, trans fats, caffeine, and high fructose corn syrup; all of these increase insulin resistance (e.g., sugar diabetes).
- Pasta, unless protein enriched
- Bread

Choose:

- Eat a high protein breakfast every morning. It will stabilize your blood sugar and get you off to a good start. Try making *protein* the focus of each meal. It kicks your metabolism into higher gear.
- All meats, fish, and poultry are the real "guilt-free" foods. Protein helps you handle insulin better. It builds muscle and repairs tissue, which are essential for staying lean and preventing diabetes. Protein also helps the production of neurotransmitters.
- Choose colorful vegetables that are low glycemic.
- Choose colorful fruits, such as berries and fruits you can eat with the skin on.

- Snack on nuts and seeds. They are a good source of protein and contain Omega 3s and Omega 9s
- Drink purified water (ounces equal to half your weight in pounds)

For a comprehensive discussion and list of glycemic index foods, see the website www.mendosa.com.

I also recommend cardiologist Stephen Sinatra's online newsletter "Heart, Health and Nutrition" at www.heartMDinstitute.com; in particular, his discussion about the five "biggest cholesterol myths." It's not all bad news!

Healthy Eating,
William H. Lee, M.D.

Appendix

Toxic Nation

Today's stealth killers are toxic heavy metals and other chemicals that accumulate in the body throughout our lifetime. In the past century, with our growing high-tech industry and chemists, we have managed to create more than 80,000 chemicals. In the United States alone, in 1994 we released into our fragile environment 2.2 million pounds of chemical toxins. We are contaminating everything: air, water, soil, plants, animals, our entire food chain, ourselves. Among the worst toxins are mercury, lead, cadmium, arsenic, pesticides, insecticides, dioxins, phthalates, furans, and PCBs.

How Bad Is It?

Most of us have between 400-800 toxic, carcinogenic, endocrine-disrupting, gene-damaging chemicals *stored* in our body, especially in the fat cells. It is estimated that as many 25 percent of the U.S. population suffer from heavy metal poisoning to some extent.

It seriously concerns me to think what this is doing to our progeny. Fetuses *now* growing in-utero are contaminated with hundreds of foreign chemicals. It is estimated that 630,000 of the four million babies now being born in the U.S. are at risk of brain damage and learning difficulties, due to mercury exposure alone (the level of mercury in the fetal circulation is 1.7 times higher than in the mother). *Could this be part of the epidemic of autism and/or attention deficit disorder? Could heavy metal poisoning be the underlying cause of the cancer epidemic in the U.S.?*

According to the Columbia University School of Public Health, 95 percent of cancer is caused by poor nutrition and environmental toxicity. It is more than just cancer. These toxic chemicals are direly affecting our neurological, endocrine, and immunological systems.

Toxicity leads to chronic health problems such as cognitive defects, mood changes, and neurologic illnesses; including autism, changes in libido, reproductive dysfunction, glucose dysregulation, immune dysfunction, autoimmunity, asthma, and allergies.

Mercury is the most destructive; and we are building coal-fired power plants all over the U.S. As the coal burns, mercury is discharged through the smoke stacks. Mercury is a deadly neurotoxin that is causing psychological, neurological, enzymatic, and immunological disorders.

The problem with heavy metals, such as mercury and lead, is that they are extremely difficult to remove from the body. The growing accumulation quickly overwhelms the body's natural detoxification pathways, resulting in severe symptoms or one or more chronic debilitating diseases. Despite the government's list of *safe* levels of these toxins, there really is no safe level of exposure to any of these toxic chemicals.

Furthermore, experts in the field of heavy-metal detoxification state that for each equivalent of stored toxins, there is an equal amount of pathogenic microorganisms in the body. Thus, the presence of stored toxins causes immune-system deficiency (dysregulation); which supports the growth of pathogens like bacteria, viruses, yeast, and parasites — and the body's own immune cells are incapacitated by the heavy metals.

This has led to the term "Toxic Body Burden" (TBB) in reference to toxic heavy metals, synthetic chemicals, and pathogens that accumulate in the body. Hence, retaining and restoring vibrant health requires an effective approach that can detoxify the toxic substances, while also eliminating the infectious microorganisms.

A Functional Medicine principal is that there exists a "web-like relationship" among all systems (immunological, neurological, gastrointestinal, circulatory, respiratory, endocrine, and detoxification); that there are relationships between the environment and genetic responses, and that we can develop programs to reliably reflect the needs of patients. This requires that we walk a broader path than the traditional model of single-factor causations, disease declension, pharmacologic and surgical treatments.

Recently, we have learned that health is directly affected by the energetics of biochemistry and genetics; which, without appropriate intervention, can eventuate into disease. David Jones, editor of "Detoxification: A Clinical Monograph," wrote, "Detoxification as a fundamental process of homeodynamic balance expends the greatest percentage of biochemical resources in the energy budget" of the human. Every molecule with which we come into contact has to be dealt with in order to chemically turn it into something we either can use or rid the body of the potential danger. He added, "When this complex process proceeds appropriately, the interplay between environment and internal milieu secures a greater probability of well being for the individual; when imbalanced, the whole system can be seriously affected. An individual's ability to detoxify substances to which he or she is exposed is of critical importance to their health."

So What Can Be Done About It?

Broadly, regarding the body's natural detoxification process, David Jones, Chief Editor of *The Textbook of Functional Medicine,* wrote, "The complex systems of the detoxification enzymes generally function adequately to minimize the potential damage from xenobiotics (substances foreign to the body whether the source is external [e.g. toxic chemicals from our environment] or internal [e.g.

food or drug byproducts not properly detoxified and eliminated]). Dysfunction and disease may occur when these systems are overloaded or not functioning adequately. These puzzling diseases include such things as chronic fatigue syndrome, fibromyalgia, multiple chemical sensitivities, possibly chronic neurologic diseases and many types of cancer (caused by polyaromatic hydrocarbons and asbestos)."

Discussing some chemistry is essential to help explain how the body's natural detoxification process takes place. As discussed in chapter 4, "Impaired Natural Detoxification," there are two phases, and the proper functioning of both is essential; because the reactive intermediate metabolites produced during *Phase I* may be more harmful or toxic than the original toxin. So, both phases must function in balance; because the amounts and types of steroids, fatty acids, and other endogenous molecules involved in cellular communication can be greatly influenced by a compromised detoxification status. Following is the science on these two phases:

The *Phase I* processes (cytochromes P450) are: oxidation, reduction, hydrolysis, hydration, and dehalogenation. The *Phase II* processes (conjugation reactions) are: glutathione conjugation, sulfation, glucuronidation, methylation, acetylation, and amino acid conjugation.

Chemical components that *induce* the *Phase I* detoxification process are, for example, cigarette smoke (polycyclic hydrocarbons), charbroiled meats (aryl amines), and some medications (e.g., Phenobarbital for epilepsy). *Phase II* activity is *induced* by many of the compounds in flavonoids (in fruits and vegetables); ellagic acid in red-grapes skin; and cruciferous vegetables (brassica family; cabbage, bok choy, broccoli, Brussels sprouts), garlic oil, rosemary, and soy.

In general, the increase in the Phase II of the body's natural detoxification process helps to promote and maintain a healthy balance between the two phases. This may be why fruits and vegetables protect against many cancers. Phase II reactions require cofactors (that must be replenished through dietary sources), plus energy in the form of ATP (comes from the Krebs Cycle, in which we convert sugar or fat into ATP). The Phase I biotransformation allows the Phase II reactions. Both the Phase I and Phase II detoxification steps can be inhibited when there are two or more compounds competing for the same detoxifying enzyme. This can happen with an increased toxic load that overwhelms the body's systems. A common mechanism of inhibition in Phase II activities is the depletion of the necessary cofactors; sulfation, in particular. The consequence of these steps is transforming toxins into harmless excretable metabolites and increasing oxidant stress and its free radical generation.

How Can You Help Your Body Detoxify?

A Healthy Gastrointestinal (GI) Tract

The GI tract is the first point of contact for the majority of xenobiotics (toxins). Support for healthy gut mucosa is instrumental in decreasing the body's toxic load. Gut microflora (good bacteria) can induce or inhibit detoxification activities. It processes a load of antigens and xenobiotics daily. Detoxification enzymes exist in the GI tract, forming a complex set of biochemical systems to manage the load. It is a barrier to all kinds of toxins.

Watch Your Medications

Make sure you are taking only the medications you really need, according to your doctor, because medications can alter the body's natural ability to detoxify. For example, defective drug metabolizing enzymes and pathways can have variable consequences. There could be a functional overdose secondary to inefficient or inadequate elimination of a drug; or there could be a lack of efficacy of a medication secondary to increased elimination of a drug. There could be idiosyncratic reactions, giving symptoms of toxicity.

In summary, the detoxification system in humans is extensive, highly complex, and has a myriad of natural regulatory mechanisms.

Nutrition

Supporting the body's natural detoxification system can range simply from good nutritional intake to supplementation with antioxidants. A therapeutic nutritional program should remove foods and beverages that are likely to contain toxins, food allergens, or an antigenic challenge to the body. The program also must meet basic nutritional needs, including adequate high-value protein and increased amounts of nutrients that function as cofactors for the two enzymatic phases.

Lastly, the body needs adequate hydration with purified water to aid the elimination of toxins. A complete detoxification program also may require optimizing the body's composition by decreasing the fat stores (where toxins are mostly stored).

Nutrients Required for the Body's Biochemical Pathways

- *Sulfation* reactions require vitamin A, adequate protein intake, and adequate sources of dietary sulfur (some amino acids, some foods such as garlic and onions).

- *Glucuronidation* reactions require magnesium. As this is a cell membrane-bound enzyme system, the integrity of the bi-lipid layer is important; meaning, omega 3 fatty acids (fish oil) is a key nutrient.

- *Glutathione* reactions are some of the most crucial in the deactivation of xenobiotics. Synthesis of these cofactors requires sufficient vitamins B_6 and B_{12}, magnesium, and folate; the brassica family vegetables (cabbage, Brussels sprouts, broccoli); and cofactor amino acids (glycine or taurine).

Nutrients That Support Detoxifying the Body

- *Sodium sulfate:* Sulfation reactions.

- *Amnio acid cofactors:* Glycine, taurine, methionine, cysteine, n-acetyl carnitine.

- *N-acetyl cysteine* (NAC, the "master antioxidant"): Amino acid that contributes significantly to glutathione synthesis.

- *Glutathione:* Xenobiotic detoxifer and antioxidant.

- *Antioxidant vitamins and minerals:* Vitamins A, mixed carotenes, C, mixed E, zinc, manganese, and selenium.

- *Flavonoids:* Naringenin (in grapefruit juice), rutin and quercetin (in tea, onions, some citrus foods), tangeretin and nobeletin (in orange juice).

- *Monoterpnoids:* Limonene and mormilin (citrus foods; induces phase II glutathione and glucuronidation activities).

- *Curcumin:* Active component in the spice turmeric; potent antioxidant, anti-inflammatory, anti-mutagen (anti-cancerous); induces glutathione.

- *Forskolin:* Enhances lypolysis, by increasing cyclic AMP.

- *Indole-3-carbinol:* In brassica foods (cabbage, brussel sprouts, broccoli); enhances Phase II glutathione pathways.

- *Rosemary:* Contains the flavonoids carnosol, carnosic acid, rosmanol, and ursolic acid which have high antioxidant activity. These are part of the polyphenols.

Detoxify Estrogen

Estrogen must be detoxified (changed into another form) so that neither women nor men get too much nor a prolonged activation of it in the body. While this was discussed in the Women's Guide, we are elaborating on it further here because it is so vital to avoiding cancer.

Estrogen goes through the Phase I and Phase II conversions of the molecule. If the metabolite of Phase I detoxification is not subsequently completed by going through the Phase II detoxification step, the middle metabolite can do more harm; whereas, Phase II totally inactivates estrogen so that it is harmless in terms of promoting cancer. There are tests that can be done on blood or urine to determine how well or how poorly you are detoxifying estrogen. See the footnote below for the science on this.[5]

The risk of breast cancer can be reduced by taking DIM (phase 1) and a "methylator" (phase 2) like methyl-cobalamine (vitamin B), methyl-folate, SAMe, MSM, or tri-methyl glycine. All of these are available in health-food stores.

Additionally, when thinking about reducing breast cancer, there is growing evidence that bioidentical progesterone (used to balance estrogen) also reduces one's risk of breast cancer (see EPIC study discussion in the Women's Guide). It appears that the synthetic progestins (progesterone look-a-likes) act differently in the body and are likely the cause of increased risk of breast cancer reported for those taking HRT.

---

[5] Phase I estrogen detoxification is all about the process *hydroxylation.* This simply means that a "hydroxyl group" (-OH) is added to the estrogen molecule. This process can be aided by DIM (di-indole methane) or I3C (Indole-3-carbonol). DIM is simply two I3Cs attached to one another. I3C is a compound found in cruciferous vegetables (broccoli, brussel sprouts, cauliflower, cabbage, kail, mustard greens); it is difficult or impossible to eat enough of these vegetables to provide enough I3C to the body.

Phase II estrogen detoxification is all about the process *methylation,* which adds a "methyl group" (-CH$_3$) to the molecule. The problem here is that as many as 40%-50% of Americans have a minor genetic defect (SNP, pronounced "snip," or Single Nucleotide Polymorphism) which makes those people poor methylators. This is why prenatal vitamins contain 1 mg of folic acid and B vitamins. Poor methylation in a pregnant mother can be related to an increased risk of a "neural tube defect" in the baby. Poor methylation in any female can result in poor Phase II detoxification of estrogen; which, theoretically, increases the risk of breast cancer. Part of the reason for "inheriting" an increased risk for breast cancer may be through this mechanism of poor methylation.

One must be careful in reading about progesterones, however, to be clear whether the author is talking about *bioidentical* progesterone *or* progestin (provera, methoxyprogesterone acetate, norethindrone). Many authors carelessly call progestins progesterone — when they are nothing alike, as discussed thoroughly in the Women's Guide.

The complexities of the body's detoxification system and an individual's ability to detoxify substances ingested suggests that a single test to fully assess one's detoxification status is not possible. The standard test today to evaluate your body is to measure the metabolites in your urine, blood, or saliva; this test takes into account the myriad factors that influence your body's detoxification activity.

Other Factors

Periodically check your liver function, through blood analysis. Because the majority of the body's detoxification process occurs in the liver, one would expect that impairment of normal liver function (due to alcoholic disease, fatty liver disease, or hepatocarcinomas) could lead to lower detoxification activity in general.

Several other factors also influence the expression and resultant activity of many detoxification enzymes; such as, age, gender, and disease influences.

In addition, be aware of your genetic history, if you can, because some versions of gene encoding (genetic polymorphisms) can affect one's ability to metabolize xenobiotics. This means, you can have "slow metabolizers" and "fast metabolizers."

Testing

The presence of toxic elements and heavy metals also can be tested (e.g., mercury, lead, arsenic, cadmium, aluminum, nickel). However, these toxic metals are largely undetected by standard laboratory analyses. Therefore, the recommended test is an elemental hair analysis or a DMSA challenge test that releases bound heavy metals from the body so they then can be measured in the urine.

In summary, toxins are abundant, ubiquitous, and dangerous to our human existence. I believe that total toxic burden is being exceeded in most of us. This burden is overwhelming our health, by decreasing the normal functions of our immunological, endocrine, circulatory, and neurological systems.

The answer is to avoid toxins as much as possible. Plus, bolster the body's natural detoxification system by providing the very necessary nutrition, exercise, sleep, and supplementation.

Appendix

A Perspective on Spiritual Aging

Excerpt from Rev. Jane Anne Ferguson's Article

The greatest opportunity of aging is to remember that we are "spiritual beings having a spiritual experience in a human body."[6]

Aging is an opportunity to harvest the wisdom of our lives . . . and to leave a legacy that contributes to the healing of the world. As I grow older, with more knowledge and hopefully more wisdom, I am experiencing at deeper and deeper levels that my mind and body live within, and are embraced by, the energy of my spirit. As I write this letter, I am one month short of fifty-five. Aging is staring me in the face.

I have been an age management/hormone patient of Dr. Lee's for almost five years. I first came to him because peri-menopause was wrecking my mind! I couldn't think anymore. I couldn't organize my

---

[6] John O'Donahue, *Anam Cara; A Celtic Book of Wisdom.* (New York, NY: Harper Perennial, 2004), 194.

thoughts as I tried to parent two teenagers after divorce, take care of my house, and meet the needs of my fifty-five to sixty-hour a week job as a parish minister. Oh, *and* I wanted to lose weight to feel good enough about myself, to begin dating again after twenty-seven years of marriage.

The hormone therapy was miraculous and continues to be. It helps to restore my clear thinking and balances my body chemistry; I have the energy to eat well and exercise often. It also gives me a sense of physical sensuality I never had before.

With this, I have had the courage to come to terms in my mind, heart, soul, and body with those leftover, nagging body-image issues from my teens and twenties: To love myself for myself. To love my body as a temple of my spirit and a reflection of divine, universal love. As I care for my body and my mind, through the healthy practices of nutrition, exercise and hormone therapy, I have the foundation for the soul work of aging.

Moving into our Elder years, the second half of life, can be a gloriously freeing experience — if we approach it from love rather than fear. It is not without its challenges. It requires caring for ourselves in ways we never did. It asks that we nurture the precious resources that are our body, mind and spirit — resources that reflect the divine light within. As we age, perhaps what we have most yet to discover is our own soul as friend.

Aging should produce Elders, not old people. Age Management practices are not a quest for eternal youth. They are a foundation for transformation. As we stand at the edge of this new quest, we have the opportunity for the deepest form of transformation. Aging is a time of harvesting all the "failures" and successes of our lives, all the events and memories, painful and joyful. We have the opportunity to see this time not as a demise of the body, but as the harvest of our soul.

Devoting our attention to our soul, embracing our life anew, even as we embrace our journey toward death, oddly enough brings new energy and purpose. We are given a new question: What shall we leave with this world to make it a better place?

It is often said that getting older is not for the faint of heart. It requires stamina, perseverance, and courage. These are concrete tools for becoming our own soul friend, for harvesting our life and facing death, and for discovering the legacy we want to leave with the world.

Healthy eldering (sage-ing) requires that we be willing to contemplate, engage our shadow side, forgive ourselves and others, reclaim our soul, and build a bridge of new growth. Dr. Lee's Age Management protocol is allowing me to do this. His Age Management protocol has provided me a foundation of energy and greater health to be able to address my deeper issues of life.

Letting go, blessing memories, people and objects has allowed me to harvest the wisdom of my many rich experiences. Engaging in forgiveness of myself and others has allowed me to reframe the "failures" of my life into opportunities for growth and learning. To be my own soul friend has freed me from the past.

I have come to appreciate the art of contemplation and how it contributes to my whole being. The art of contemplation is intertwined with the art of solitude. Sitting to breathe and quiet my mind does not come naturally to me. I am a feeler and a doer. I rise each morning with swirling thoughts of all that must be accomplished.

Learning the grounding practice of connecting to Spirit and to my spirit through quiet sitting and breathing, as well as through journaling, gives me the courage daily to age more wisely — in all aspects of my physical routines and soulful development. It connects me to the bigger picture of my life. It reminds me that I am first and foremost a spiritual being. I am divine energy connected to the Divine. I am a beloved Child of God. I am a part of God.

This daily contemplation and solitude puts all my concerns of work and personal life into perspective. It reminds me that I do not have to be driven by the worry and fears of my life. I can live in the Heart of God and be connected to the Source through my Higher Self, my soul. Through this practice, I am my own soul friend, day by day.

Appendix

Progesterone and Breast Cancer Risk

This is very new information that most people, even doctors, don't know about yet. I feel it is critical for women's awareness to share it. Even though in places this content gets a little heavy on the science, I feel it is best, for your health, to be informed and up-to-date on the latest results of studies published regarding breast cancer risks.

There is tremendous confusion regarding progesterone and breast cancer risk. Even among doctors of medicine, the confusion remains. It seems to stem from the hysteria caused by the Women's Health Initiative (WHI) 2002 news release that received enormous and unusual media attention. *Here are the facts:*

We now know the difficulties in interpreting the findings in the WHI study. It involved 161,000 women who either participated in a set of clinical trials, to test preventive measures for heart disease, fractures, breast and colorectal cancer; or were part of a large double-blind, placebo-controlled study. The study participants received either conjugated equine estrogen (CEE) 0.625 mg, or placebo in the estrogen-alone arm of the study. In the estrogen-plus-progestin arm, the study participants received CEE 0.625 mg plus medroxyprogesterone acetate (MPA) 2.5 mg or placebo.

Important facts: We now know that the WHI 2002 study participants were older (average age 63, when they first started hormone therapy; as many age 70+ as age 50), overweight (average BMI 28.5, 30 were obese), and 50 percent were past or current smokers.

The estrogen-alone arm of the WHI study was stopped prematurely in February 2004, after approximately seven years, because of the increased risk of stroke and no reduction in the risk of coronary heart disease. This estrogen-alone arm was carried out in forty clinical centers, seeing 10,739 generally healthy women ages 50-79, who had undergone a hysterectomy. The estrogen-plus-progestin trial was stopped after 5.6 years, in July 2002, because of an observed increased risk of breast cancer (this is what was hit so hard by the confused media, with all of the fanfare and bias). This combination therapy was also observed to increase the risk of heart disease.

Breast cancer developed in 245 of the 8,506 women who had been randomized to the estrogen-plus-progestin group; and in 185 of the 8,102 women randomized to the placebo group. Of these cancers, 349 were invasive. The WHI conclusions published in the *Journal of the American Medical Association* (*JAMA*) in 2002 were based upon the group of invasive cancers. The conclusion was that there is an increased risk of breast cancer due to CEE + MPA. Statistically, however, there would be eight additional cases of invasive breast cancer out of every 10,000 women in one year.

Following the release of this information, as many as 70 percent of women around the world stopped taking their hormones for fear of breast cancer, heart disease, stroke, and blood clots. Now nine years later, cutting-edge doctors who have been studying the recent literature know that all of these risks are explainable — and are not truly risks.

This new information has been very slow to reach both the medical community and the lay public. Some of the continuation of the panic comes from follow-up information released to the media, like the following:

In February 2009, in the *New England Journal of Medicine,* Rowan T. Chlebowski, M.D., Ph.D., and other WHI scientists, examined data to help explain why there had been a drop in the rates of breast cancer since the release of the WHI report. They confirmed that the risk of breast cancer associated with estrogen-plus-progestin use goes down significantly once the hormones are stopped. He and others, however, ignored the fact that many women have been turning to bioidentical hormones for their treatment of menopause and the enhancement of their quality of life. In fact, in the face of this increase in bioidentical hormone use, *breast cancer rates dropped!*

Additionally, it has been observed that about 5-7 percent of estrogen-alone participants in the WHI 2002 study stopped taking their pills (CEE or placebo) each year. More than half (54%) were no longer taking pills by year seven. This drop-out rate would invalidate many studies; but the WHI continues to publish its old, disproven finding despite the enormous drop-out rate.

On April 12, 2006, the final report from the WHI of all breast cancers diagnosed before the estrogen-alone trial was stopped, was published in *JAMA*. There was an average 7.1 years of follow-up from 237 invasive breast cancers. There was a 20 percent *lower* risk of invasive breast cancer in the estrogen-alone group, compared to the placebo group. This reduction was not quite statistically significant, although some statisticians proclaim this as statistically significant. The details are: 104 cases of invasive breast cancer in the CEE group (28 cases per 10,000 women per year), compared to 133 cases in the placebo group (34 cases per 10,000 women per year). At least we can say, there is *no* increased risk of breast cancer for seven years if medroxyprogesterone acetate (MPA) (Provera) is *not* used.

The conclusion stated by Stanford University's Marcia Stefanick, Ph.D., the study's lead author and chair of the WHI Steering Committee, said, "What is clear now is that, overall, postmenopausal women without a uterus who choose to take estrogen-alone do not have an increased breast cancer risk, at least over the first 7 years of treatment."

Jacques Rossouw, M.D., chief of the NHLBI Women's Health Initiative Branch, stated, "The increased risk of breast cancer found in women taking combined hormones may be due to the effects of progestin – when it is combined with estrogen."

In addition, women in the CEE group had a 33 percent *lower* risk of breast cancer, compared to those in the placebo group; and CEE appears to reduce the risk of ductal breast cancer, which is the most common form. Another way to state this is: *Progestin, particularly MPA, **increases** breast cancer risk.*

In April 2007, Jacques Rossouw, M.D., published in *JAMA* his follow-up to the WHI report. He singled out from the original study group only those women who were within ten years of menopause. In this subgroup of women, the increased incidence of breast cancer was only 1 or 2 out every 10,000 women. To me, this is a very small number. Especially when one considers, that Rossouw also pointed out that in this younger subgroup of women, the *decreased* incidence of heart disease was 35 percent (3,500 out of every 10,000 women). These numbers *are* overwhelmingly favorable for the use of CEE (Premarin) and MPA (Provera).

Furthermore, we now have the French E3N EPIC (European Prospective Investigation into Cancer and Nutrition) prospective cohort study for further guidance, published in January 2008 in *Breast Cancer Research and Treatment*. Because it is a European study, it has not received as much attention as the American WHI 2002 report.

However, this 2008 study is well done and has very good numbers to support it.

Initiated in 1990, half a million women were invited to participate in the French EPIC study; 98,995 volunteered to participate, including 80,377 post-menopausal women. They were ages 40-65, living in metropolitan France, mostly teachers, all insured with a large French insurer. Invasive breast cancer cases were identified through biennial self-administered questionnaires completed from 1990 to 2002.

Follow up on this French study revealed 2,354 cases of invasive breast cancer occurred among 80,377 postmenopausal women (average 8.1 postmenopausal years). Compared to women who had never used hormones, use of estrogen-alone was associated with a significant 1.29-fold increased risk (95% confidence interval 1.02-1.65). Only 1.3 percent of the women had taken conjugated equine estrogen (CEE); most had taken estradiol, and mostly transdermal.

The association of breast cancer to estrogen-progestagen combinations varied greatly with the type of progestagen. The relative risk for estrogen-dydrogesterone combination was 1.16 (0.94-1.43); whereas, the estrogen-other progestagens combination was 1.69 (1.50-1.91). *However, the relative risk of breast cancer for estrogen-progesterone was only 1.00 (0.83-1.22). A relative risk of 1.00 means there is no increased risk at all.*

Thus, once again, the choice of progesterone vs. progestin in combination with estrogen is critically important. The media, and even some M.D.s, have been loosely using the words progesterone and progestin interchangeably in their reports. The media is confused, and confusing. And doctors have been misled by the incorrect usage of terms and an incorrect dissemination of information.

The conclusion remains: "Combinations containing micronized progesterone appeared to be associated with a significantly lower breast cancer risk than those containing synthetic progestins."

In 2007, Wood et al. published in *Breast Cancer Research Treatment,* comparing the effects of estradiol given with either MPA (progestin) or micronized bioidentical progesterone, on risk biomarkers for breast cancer in twenty-six postmenopausal cynomolgus monkeys. In this randomized crossover trial, they found that estradiol and MPA had resulted in significantly increased proliferation of at least 30 percent in lobular and ductal breast epithelium. This is consistent with breast cancer risk estimates from many clinical trials. This was measured by genetic Ki67 expression, and cyclin B1, and estrogen receptor expression activity (ER alpha, PGR, TFF1).

Wood reported: "Compared to placebo treatment, lobular proliferation was 99% greater after estradiol (E2) (P = 0.09), 58% greater after E2 + Progesterone (P4) (P = 0.47), and 194% greater after E2 + MPA (P = 0.009). Ductal proliferation was also significantly higher after E + MPA treatment (+544%, P = 0.006 vs placebo) but not E2 (-38%, P = 0.80) or E2 + progesterone (+75%, P = 0.72)."

This study supports that, when combined with estrogen, progesterone may have a *safer* risk profile in the breast. Progesterone given either orally or intravaginally induces less stimulation in the post menopausal breast than does MPA. Serum concentrations of 3-5 ng/ml are the minimum required for endometrial suppression. The minimum concentration needed for breast protection has not been established.

Wood's conclusion was, "The addition of the synthetic progestin MPA to postmenopausal estrogen therapy significantly increases breast cancer risk. These findings suggest that oral micronized progesterone has a more favorable effect on risk biomarkers for postmenopausal breast cancer than medroxyprogesterone acetate (MPA)."

In 1998, Jean-Michel Foidart, M.D., Ph.D., published in *Fertility and Sterility* his work of giving forty postmenopausal women hormones for two weeks prior to breast surgery, wherein breast tissue was obtained and could be sent to the lab for analysis. Women used a gel applied to both breasts daily for fourteen days prior to their plastic surgery. The gels were one of four: (1) estradiol 1.5 mg.d, (2) progesterone 25 mg/d, (3) estradiol 1.5 mg/d + progesterone 25 mg/d, and (4) placebo. From the breast tissue and blood tests, Foidart determined estradiol and progesterone levels, and quantitated proliferating cell nuclear antigen expression. His findings were that estradiol significantly stimulates the proliferation of normal breast cells and that progesterone dramatically limits the proliferation of breast cells in women.

In 2003, Henk Franke and Istvan Vermes published their European study from the Netherlands in *Maturitas, The European Menopause Journal*. It compared proliferation vs. apoptosis in estrogen receptor (ER) positive human breast cancer cells when given various different progestogens and estradiol in vitro. Franke and Vermes showed that, in vitro, not all progestogens act equally on breast cancer cells (some progestogens, MPA and norethisterone acetate [NETA] alone, or combined with E2, stimulate proliferation of breast cancer cells; progesterone alone, or combined with E2, induces apoptosis). They wrote: "The balance between programmed cell death (apoptosis) and cell proliferation determines the tumor growth rate, and any alteration between these two factors may be a key element for the uncontrolled expansion of malignant tumors."

Similarly, in 1998, Bent Formby, Ph.D. published in the *Annals of Clinical and Laboratory Science* more information regarding progesterone and apoptosis. Progesterone inhibits the proliferation of normal breast epithelial cells in vivo, as well as breast cancer cells in vitro. He investigated p53 and bcl-2, because they genetically control the apoptotic process. He found a 90 percent inhibition of cell proliferation with T47-D breast cancer cells after exposure to progesterone. After twenty-four hours of exposure to progesterone, the expression of T47-D cancer cells of bcl-2 was down-regulated, and that of p53 was up-regulated. These results demonstrate that progesterone exhibits a strong antiproliferative effect on two breast cancer cell lines. Formby wrote, "The results of our work confirm the fact that the levels of bcl-2 and p53 expression are inversely regulated by progesterone concomitantly with induced apoptosis and inhibition of growth. Progesterone inhibits proliferation of breast cancer cells up to 90% in T47-D breast cancer cells."

In 2002, Alkhalaf et al. published similar findings in the *European Journal of Cancer Prevention*. They showed that progesterone inhibits the proliferation of normal breast epithelial cells in vivo, as well as breast cancer cells in vitro. They showed that growth inhibition of breast cancer cells by progesterone is due to the induction of cell differentiation, and not apoptosis.

In 1981, Cowan et al. published in the *American Journal of Epidemiology* a study of breast cancer incidence in women with a history of progesterone deficiency. He studied 1,083 women as to their cause of infertility. During a thirty-three year follow-up, it was found that progesterone-deficient women had 5.4 times the risk of premenopausal breast cancer, and a ten-fold increase in death from all malignant neoplasms.

In 1995, Chang et al. published his work in *Fertility and Sterility,* a double-blind randomized study in which he had topically applied progesterone, estradiol, or a combination of the two, or placebo, daily for ten to thirteen days, mimicking the luteal phase. In surgically biopsied breast epithelium, he showed that the number of cycling epithelial cells increased with estradiol. However, that progesterone significantly decreased the number of cycling epithelial cells. In other words, progesterone reduced estradiol-induced proliferation. Chang concluded, "It indicates that natural progesterone replacement can prevent normal breast epithelium from transforming into estradiol-induced hyperplasia."

In 1990, Barrat et al. published in *Gynecologic and Obstetrical Biology of Reproduction* his findings that sustained levels of progesterone in breast tissue greater than ten days decreased mitotic activity in normal breast tissue. Thus, just like in the endometrium, progesterone controls the human breast epithelial cell cycle during a normal fourteen-day luteal phase. To the contrary, some synthetic progestins, especially in oral contraceptives, have been reported to stimulate proliferation of breast cancer cells (Jeng et al., 1992, *Cancer Research*; Jordan, 1993, *Cancer*).

Conclusions

Conflicting evidence exists as to the association of estrogen and breast cancer. First, conjugated equine estrogen does not appear to cause breast cancer, as reported by the WHI estrogen-alone arm. However, the 1999 French EPIC study shows us that estradiol alone may increase breast cancer 29 percent. There may be some modulating factor among the ten estrogens in conjugated equine estrogens.

It is becoming quite clear that the choice of micronized progesterone, over other progestins, has distinct advantages. Not only does progesterone inhibit breast cancer, especially compared to progestins like medroxyprogesterone acetate (MPA), but it also lowers lipids and it dilates coronary blood vessels. The breast cancer inhibition was shown very well in the French EPIC study.

The other studies described here reinforce this concept, by showing genetic Ki67 expression in monkeys. Foidart's 1998 findings were that estradiol significantly stimulates the proliferation of normal breast cells, and that progesterone dramatically limits the proliferation of breast cells in women. Franke's 2003 study showed that progestins stimulate proliferation of breast cancer cells; progesterone alone, or combined with E2 induce apoptosis. Formby's 1998 study showed that progesterone inhibits proliferation of breast cancer cells up to 90 percent in T47-D breast cancer cells. Alkhalaf's 2002 study showed that growth inhibition of breast cancer cells by progesterone is due to the induction of cell differentiation and not apoptosis. Cowan's 1981 study found that progesterone deficient women had 5.4 times the risk of premenopausal breast cancer, and a ten-fold increase in death from all malignant neoplasms. Plus, we have multiple authors speaking about the benefits of sustained progesterone.

Carefully read these issues, so that you don't promulgate the ignorance regarding progestins vs. real progesterone. There is a huge difference to your health.

Bottom line: Progesterone is safe and effective. It allows increased protection against breast cancer.

Appendix

The Misleading 2002 WHI Report

The 2002 Women's Health Initiative (WHI) study — along with the U.S. Preventive Services Task Force (USPSTF), American College of OB-Gyn (ACOG), and North American Menopause Society (NAMS) — got it wrong.

They recommended against the "routine use of combined estrogen and progestin for the prevention of chronic conditions in postmenopausal women." They recommended against the "routine use of unopposed estrogen for the prevention of chronic conditions in postmenopausal women who have had a hysterectomy." The edict, or general rule of thumb from these organizations was: "Give the lowest dose possible for the shortest period of time."

Not one single study supports these statements. If estrogen and the other hormones were unhealthy or dangerous, I would agree that the lowest dose possible for the shortest period of time would be solid advice. However, what I am telling you in this book is that estrogen is *very* good for you!

Each woman needs the appropriate dose for her individual body, determined by regular blood tests, for the rest of her life. Just thinking logically, how could something important for your normal functioning, that your own body produces forty to fifty years, suddenly become bad for you? Hormones do not become harmful or bad for us — as long as they are *bioidentical.*

It is important to remember that the Women's Health Initiative "randomized controlled trial" used only horse-derived estrogen and artificial progesterone. The USPSTF found that "combined estrogen and progestin is associated with both benefits and harms. The benefits include reduced fracture risk [good evidence] and colorectal cancer risk [fair evidence].... However, combined estrogen and progestin has no beneficial effect on coronary artery disease (CHD) and may even increase risk [good evidence]." They also wrote: "Other deleterious effects include increased risk for breast cancer [good evidence], stroke [fair evidence], cholecystitis [fair evidence], dementia [fair evidence] and lower global cognitive function [fair evidence]."

However, the following statement is incomprehensible to me: "Because of insufficient evidence, the USPSTF could not assess the effects of combined estrogen and progestin on the incidence of ovarian cancer, mortality from breast cancer or CHD, or all-cause mortality."

The WHI study authors did note that the combined risks for CHD and breast cancer that can be attributed to hormone therapy are low. On the basis of their results, for example, there would be seven more cases of CHD events [<0.01%], eight more strokes [<0.01%], eight more pulmonary emboli [<0.01%], and eight more cases of invasive breast cancer [<0.01%] each year for every 10,000 women. Conversely, the absolute risk reduction for every 10,000 women each year would be six fewer cases of colorectal cancer [<0.01%] and five fewer hip fractures [<0.01%].

I also totally disagree with this statement: "The USPSTF concluded that the harmful effects of combined estrogen and progestin are likely to exceed the chronic disease prevention benefits in most women."

Yet the following statement is true regarding the effects of estrogen: "The balance of benefits and harms for a woman are influenced by her personal preferences, risks for specific chronic diseases, and the presence of menopausal symptoms."

Yes, a shared decision-making approach to preventing chronic diseases in peri-menopausal women and post-menopausal women involves consideration of *individual* risk factors and preferences when selecting effective interventions to reduce the risks of fractures, heart disease, and cancer.

For additional information and a more comprehensive discussion on the WHI study and more recent studies, see "The Women's Guide" in the section on estrogen.

Appendix

Brain Memory

I asked Michael Hickey for a chapter on measuring memory. He is the co-founder of WAVi, along with David Oakley, a company for which I am the medical director. Of Hickey's numerous new medical products, the most famous is the Pulse Oximeter, which is used in every ER, ICU, OR, etc.

WAVi is an innovation of EEG technology intended for measuring memory and calculating variance from normative to aid in differentiating dementia from Alzheimer's, anxiety, depression, and obsessive-compulsive disorder. This new product will be out in 2012. I'll have one of the very first in my office.

The following chapter is about memory and how we can use an EEG to measure memory. It was written for Michael Hickey by Travis Moe who works at the company. The information comes from Michael as well as David Joffe, the WAVi biomedical engineer who created the Pulse Oximeter with Michael Hickey and Scott Wilbur.

The New WA Vi Clinic Brain Scanner

Nearly 100 million Americans face age-related health declines, and we find ourselves in the midst of a healthcare crisis. Direct and indirect costs of mental diseases, ranging from mild cognitive impairment (MCI) to Alzheimer's, amount to hundreds of billions of dollars each year, a number that fails to account for the enormous emotional cost on the victims of these diseases and their loved ones.

All current solutions meant to solve this crisis (e.g., brain scans, eye exams, spinal taps, psychometric tests) have failed due to an inability to provide early enough detection and preventative treatment during the stages when these diseases can be treated most effectively. These failures are byproducts of limited methodologies, lack of accessibility, and because the technologies are far too expensive to be utilized *before* symptoms appear, at which point the diseases are already very advanced.

The paradox of early detection, as it is currently attempted, is that scans of patients cannot be justified financially until there are strong enough proofs of the possibility of a disease; however, once these proofs are observed, it no longer counts as "early detection." New low-cost solutions that can detect mental decline accurately and are quick and easy enough to use in routine physical exams are needed desperately.

On the research end of understanding mental health, the technology needed to quantify the rises and falls of performance due to myriads of external factors, has been around a long time; yet, the problem always has been the cost. If a researcher wanted to study the effect of running (two miles every day for two months) on the brains of patients between the ages of sixteen and forty, it might prove to be an interesting case; but it would be extremely difficult to acquire funding because the enormous cost of even such a simple study would far outweigh the perceived return on the information.

For researchers looking to track and quantify the results on the brain of any course of active treatment (e.g., exercise, meditation, hormones, biofeedback), supplemental treatment (e.g., natural herbs or pharmaceuticals) or lifestyle change (e.g., changes in diet, alcohol/caffeine consumption), no system currently exists that is cheap enough to merit conducting these potentially hugely important studies. While it can be easily assumed that improvements in a person's self-care will lead to improvements in brain functioning, what is needed is a method to prove it quantifiably and scientifically.

Imagine a man who has trouble concentrating. His friends and doctors suggest meditation. He is willing to try it for the sake of his health. After a month, he thinks he might be experiencing a slight improvement, but he's not sure. Then his daily meditation slips to once a week, then ceases altogether.

What if there was a way, in the span of a few minutes and for only a few dollars, to scan his brain once a week and to see undeniably the positive changes taking place in his brain activity due to the daily meditation? That kind of quantitative proof could be the exact thing he needs to motivate him to keep it up long enough to really make concrete improvements in his quality of life.

The Boulder, Colorado company, WAVi, has developed such a system. It is an easy-to-use desktop tool that provides the physician access to efficient and inexpensive assessments of a patient's mental-health status. It incorporates all the strengths of the expensive, sophisticated methods of brain scanning, without their limitations (cost, special facility).

The WAVi solution will make brain scanning and analysis as easy as a blood-pressure test. With an integrated wireless and portable EEG headset, with point-of-care user friendly software and cutting-edge reference tools WAVi is poised to open a whole new world of research and substantial gains in scientific understanding of the nature and progress of brain diseases and the effects of different lifestyles on brain health.

The WAVi headset measures brain activity using an EEG (electroencephalography), which relies upon a network of electrodes to detect the voltage across different locations on the scalp over the cortex of the brain. The result is a map of the amplitude of electrical activity at each scalp site, as well as maps of the relative power of the four major wave forms (delta, theta, alpha, beta) at each site and the level of electrical variance of each site against all other scalp sites.

This provides an image of coherence and symmetry within a brain's activity.

EEG is the method of brain scanning that has been in use by far the longest (the first tests on human subjects took place in the mid-1920s). Everything from the original identification of the four major wave forms, to recognition of abnormal patterns correlated with epilepsy, to major gains currently being made in recognizing the telltale biomarkers of diseases (such as Alzheimer's, autism, schizophrenia, depression, ADD) has been accomplished using EEG. Combined with a reliable normative database, EEG is easily the strongest option for determining a patient's variance from normal. At the same time, it also has the sensitivity to pick up on subtleties of change in temporal brain activity, making it ideal for conducting the WAVi studies.

The way the WAVi system works is that after a patient has been scanned through the headset, the data is transmitted wirelessly to a physician or clinician's computer; a software program automatically interprets the data using three parameters. The first and most essential is a comparison of the patient's scan to a normative value for his or her age group. Using a Gaussian bell curve demonstrating standard deviations, the software tells the physician how close to the optimal level (expected for someone of his or her age) the patient's brain is functioning. If the patient's brain activity is well outside the normal range, this is invaluable early detection. The physician knows to run further tests and begin a differential diagnosis for a disease or condition that, most likely, is not yet demonstrating symptoms. With regard to monitoring changes following a shift in lifestyle, or for researchers, these automatic comparisons against normalcy also can be used to track improvements or degradations in metrics derived from the EEG through a series of scans.

The second set of parameters that the software measures in a patient's brain activity consists of a series of physician-selected biomarkers (will increase in sophistication as the science improves). As variations in EEG wave patterns are better identified as correlating with specific disorders, the software looks for those patterns and highlights any sections of scans that might show cause for concern. The physician then knows to further examine the results of the diagnostic process.

The third and final parameter of the software does not rely on any specific biomarkers. Instead, each scan highlights variations *not yet connected* to definite biomarkers. This is an area in which the science involved may be improved greatly due to the WAVi data-processing infrastructure. Any unusual patterns not yet understood may be submitted online, through the WAVi medical network; a forum of physicians, clinicians, and researchers has been designed to foster sharing such new patterns and information. This allows discussing what these professionals might suggest, and opens the door to new veins of research.

Perhaps the most exciting aspect of this digital, web-based approach to mental assessment is that technology today enables us automatically to link scans conducted by using the WAVi system with a patient's electronic medical record (EMR). The data, attributed anonymously, then will be transmitted across the internet to the WAVi database, where the repository of scans (could quickly surpass a million) will be open-sourced freely to any researchers interested in utilizing this resource. As the most sophisticated studies currently being performed cost hundreds of thousands of dollars and usually rely on fifty subjects or fewer, it is easy to imagine how studies conducted potentially on millions of subjects, for close to no cost, could lead to an exponential explosion in the quality and depth of studies on the human brain. Most costs in brain-related scientific studies come from collecting the data alone. When that data is provided free of charge, the cost nearly vanishes. The results of all of these studies will be published openly, accessible to all physicians and clinicians — directly at the point of care on their computers, through an easily searched and analyzed WAVi Digital Library.

The major innovation provided here is in the widely accessible technology, mode of communication, and transfer of data. For example, WAVi will allow a clinician in an athletic club to scan a patient on a rigid exercise routine over the course of a year; and submit all that data, with notes and observations, to the community, in a manner similar to that of a highly trained researcher.

Also, a collection of physicians will be able to scan patients in different parts of the world *and* begin to recognize patterns in the scans, which can be discussed in the collaborative forum across the internet. For example, a researcher at a university in Switzerland may envision a comparative study of the scans of 500 residents in each of the ten largest cities in Japan and speculate as to the possible effects of the various climates and different urban centers on the functioning of people's brains. That researcher can freely access the data and submit the finds to the global community at large.

In conjunction with the creativity and capabilities of individual clinicians and researchers, supercomputers currently being developed also will play a part in brain research. With the ultra-large samplings of data funneled into a single locale will come the ability to aggregate, cross-reference, and data-mine for patterns not recognized previously due to their subtlety and complexity. Currently unforeseeable patterns may emerge through compiling vast amounts and different types of data. Innovated forms of processing may revolutionize and revitalize the use of EEG in brain health, diagnosis, and treatment.

With regards to applying these innovations to managing the aging process, that's where all the technology comes together. Not only will the normative database provide an anchor of understanding what "normal aging" actually means; it will provide markers by which to recognize a brain that is resisting the most damaging effects of getting old. The WAVi headset tracks what works and what doesn't.

More importantly, I believe we must ask ourselves what physiological "aging" really means. For the sake of argument, I define here aging as the process by which the human body gradually ceases to function at full capacity, without the biological strengths of youth and full health.

One of the great virtues of EEG is its ability to identify areas in the brain that have faltered, declined in usage, or become neglected. EEG can help to locate atrophies that have taken place over time in a human body, revealing a necessary course of treatment for that patient.

The WAVi headset allows the physician to track continuously the success of such treatments (interventions) or change tactics if something is not proving effective, as well as to inform the wider medical community of what has proven to work. Because of the highly precise and individualistic nature of a patient's EEG scan, the WAVi system allows analyzing a specific case — and tailoring an individualistic course of treatment.

The application of this kind of monitoring of the brain and age-related diseases cannot be overstated. Dementia, from its mildest form (Mild Cognitive Impairment) to its most severe form (Alzheimer's), is one of the most devastating illnesses facing the aging population. Its burdens are the psychological grief on the patients and their families, as well as the staggering cost. It is notable to mention that in 2010 the worldwide cost of dementia is estimated up to $604 billion, a cost expected to triple by 2050.[7]

Currently, the only known method of preventing dementia (few pharmaceuticals have proven useful) is a change in lifestyle following very early detection. The WAVi system provides a method of very early detection.

In addition to the clinical usage of EEG, an equally critical function of the WAVi platform is biofeedback (i.e., neurotherapy). It is no secret that one of the main causes of rapid aging is stress. It is also commonly agreed today that the best cure for stress is relaxation. What may be something of a secret is that the FDA recognizes EEG self-regulation operant *relaxation training* as a safe and effective technique for stress-reduction therapy; in fact, this is the only relaxation-training therapy for which the FDA has granted regulatory clearance. The WAVi software provides relaxation training — not only to prevent or delay the most destructive aspects of aging, but also as active neurotherapies to build competencies to compensate for some of the losses that have come with age and atrophy. Simply put, the WAVi system teaches an individual treated how to use his or her brain in new ways.

A result of the groundbreaking WAVi system, healthcare, as we know it, is currently perched on the cusp of a major change. The future of data no longer will be in proprietary data silos, kept away (except for a fee) from those who could do the most with it. The future of

---

[7] http://www.alz.co.uk/research/worldreport

mental assessment is no longer in psychometric tests or expensive brain scans (that come far too late). Large-scale data collection from all demographics (an exponentially larger amount of data than has ever existed) will be available freely to all scientists — making preventive care cheap, fast, and efficient. The future of brain-related healthcare looks very bright indeed.

Resources

Alkhalaf et al. (2002), *European Journal of Cancer Prevention.*

American Association of Anti-Aging Medicine (A4M), www.WorldHealth.net.

American College of Obstetrics and Gynecology, www.acog.org.

Barrat et al. (1990), *Gynecologic and Obstetrical Biology of Reproduction.*

Brand-Miller, Jennie, Ph.D., and Wolever, Thomas M.S., M.D., Ph.D., *The New Glucose Revolution.*

Braverman, Eric, M.D., *Younger You, The Edge Effect, The Younger (Thinner) You Diet, The Healing Nutrients Within, Male Sexual Fitness, The Amazing Way to Reverse Heart Disease*, www.pathmed.com.

Canonico, et al. (2007), *Circulation*,115: 840-845.

Cenegenics Medical Institute: Age Management Medicine, www.Cenegenics.com.

Chang et al. (1995), *Fertility and Sterility.*

Chopra, Deepak, M.D., *Grow Younger, Live Longer.*

Cowan et al. (1981), *American Journal of Epidemiology.*

Formby, Bent, Ph.D. (1998), *Annals of Clinical and Laboratory Science.*

Franke, Henk, and Vermes, Istvan (2003), *Maturitas, The European Menopause Journal.*

Graff, Cynthia Stamper, *Lean for Life: Phase 1.*

Gray, John, Ph.D., *The Mars & Venus Diet & Exercise Solution.*

Heller, Carl G., "The Male Climacteric, Its Symptomology, Diagnosis, and Treatment" in the *Journal of the American Medical Association*, 126(8): 472-477.

Holick, Michael F., M.D., Ph.D., *The Vitamin D Solution: The 3-Step Strategy to Cure Our Most Common Health Problem.*

Hotze, Steven, M.D., *Hormones, Health, and Happiness.*

Hyman, Mark, M.D., *Ultra Metabolism, The Ultra Mind Solution.*

Ignarro, Eduard, Ph.D., Nobel Prize in Medicine, *NO More Heart Disease.*

Institute for Functional Medicine, *Textbook of Functional Medicine*, www.FunctionalMedicine.org.

Klatz, Ronald, M.D., President American Academy of Anti-Aging Medicine, and Goldman, Robert, D.O., President National Academy of Sports Medicine, *The New Anti-Aging Revolution, Ten Weeks to a Younger You.*

Lee, Elizabeth, M.D., *Screaming to be Heard: Hormone Connections Women Suspect, Doctors Still Ignore.*

Life, Jeffry S. (2011), *The Life Plan, Dr. Life's Guide for Men to Great Health, Better Sex, and a Leaner Stronger Body*, Simon & Schuster.

Marks, Leonard, M.D., et al. (2006), "Effect of Testosterone Replacement Therapy on Prostate Tissue in Men with Late-onset Hypogonadism: A randomized controlled trial," *Journal of the American Medical Association.*

Mayer, Catherine (2011), *Amortality: The Pleasures and Perils of Living Agelessly.*

Morgentaler, Abraham, M.D., *Testosterone for Life.*

Northrup, Christine, M.D., *The Wisdom of Menopause.*

Null, Gary, Ph.D., *Power Aging.*

Perricone, Nicholas, M.D., *The Perricone Prescription.*

Rosedale, Ron, M.D., *The Rosedale Diet: Turn Off Your Hunger Switch.*

Rosseau, J.E., et al. (2007), *Journal of the American Medical Association,* 297:1465–1477.

Scarabin, et al., *Lancet* (2003), 362(9382): 428-32.

Schwarzbein, Diana, M.D., endocrinologist, *The Schwarzbein Principles: The Program, The Schwarzbein Principles: The Transition, The Schwarzbein Principle: The Truth About Losing Weight, Being Healthy, and Feeling Younger,* www.SchwarzbeinPrinciple.com.

Sears, Barry, Ph.D., *The Anti-Inflammation Zone.*

Shippen, Eugene, M.D., *The Testosterone Syndrome.*

Smith, Pamela Wartian, M.D., MPH, HRT: *The Answers.*

Somers, Suzanne, *The Sexy Years, Ageless, Knock Out, Breakthrough, Sexy Forever.*

Speroff, Leon, M.D., and Fritz, Marc, *Clinical Gynecologic Endocrinology and Infertility*.

Strand, Ray D., M.D., *What Your Doctor Doesn't Know About Nutritional Medicine*.

The Textbook of Functional Medicine (2005), "Detoxification and Biotransformational Imbalances."

Weil, Andrew, M.D., *Healthy Aging*.

Wilson, James L., N.D., D.C., Ph.D., *Adrenal Fatigue*.

Young, Robert, Ph.D., *The pH Miracle*.

INDEX

About the Author

D r. William H. Lee, M.D. is an OB/Gyn and specialist in Age Management and Functional Medicine, including menopause in women and andropause in men.

Born in Sioux Falls, South Dakota, he grew up in Topeka, Kansas, and graduated from the University of Kansas in 1969, with degrees in both economics and political science. He next graduated from the University of Kansas Medical School in 1973, and became Board Certified as an OB/Gyn in 1979, completing his internship and residency at the University of Southern California. He has been in private practice ever since.

After medical school, Dr. Lee began studying literature on hormones, osteoporosis, and cancer risks. His interest in hormone replacement began during medical school, when his mother suffered complications from compression fractures resulting from severe osteoporosis. In addition, Dr. Lee looked for answers for his own son's autism, which led to a clinical focus on Functional Medicine. The strenuous course "Applying Functional Medicine to Clinical Practice" was Dr. Lee's first venture into holistic medicine.

He next became Board Certified in Age Management Medicine by Cenegenics in 2004 and Anti-Aging Medicine by the American Academy of Anti-Aging Medicine in 2005.

These studies increased his knowledge in nutrition, supplementation, exercise, and stress management.

Dr. Lee lectures nationally on the value of bioidentical hormones, nutrition, exercise, and stress management. Courses he has taught include The Institute for Integrative Medicine in Las Vegas, Nevada; the Colorado Society of Clinical Specialists in Psychiatric Nursing in Breckenridge, Colorado; and the "Grand Rounds" at both the Sky Ridge and Littleton Hospitals in Colorado. Dr. Lee also regularly gives seminars locally to the lay public on topics such as menopause, andropause, nutrition, and age management.

In addition, he was the Medical Director for a ground breaking company, a ground-breaking company that has developed a device that measures memory and can differentiate dementia from Alzheimer's disease. This is especially valuable for the early detection of these diseases, something that has not been possible until now. This device will be available in doctors' offices and clinics, hopefully, in 2012, and will be posted on Dr. Lee's website www.AgeManagementMD.com.

Dr. Lee's greatest reward in life is seeing the spectacular results of his careful and deliberate care of each individual patient — because he believes in the wellness and possible prolonged longevity of the human body, by treating the whole person. At least we can make the best of all the days we have on this planet.

CPSIA information can be obtained at www.ICGtesting.com
Printed in the USA
BVOW071906060212

282308BV00001B/12/P